WEIGHT LOSS
A Rocket Science

I Dedicate this book to my Mother Kamal Bawa, Father Dr. M.M.Krishan, My Sister Nidhi Mohan Kamal, My Friends and My Teachers who made me who I am.

WEIGHT LOSS
A Rocket Science

Our believe in Eradication
Of Obesity from Mankind

DR. SUNNY BAWA

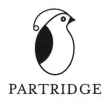

PARTRIDGE

To order additional copies of this book, contact
Partridge India
000 800 10062 62
orders.india@partridgepublishing.com

www.partridgepublishing.com/india

Contents

Introduction

Although this is the introduction to this book, to be honest, I wrote this after I finished the other parts of the book. I don't know how to start, but you've got to start to finish what you started. And I believe the same philosophy applies to your weight loss journey as well. You've got to begin somewhere, and do just a little bit and then a little bit more every day regardless of external circumstances. There will never be right circumstances to make your weight loss a reality; you have to do it for you.

The circumstances will tell you that it's your birthday, it's your anniversary, it's your friend's birthday, or it's an important day, someone died, the weather is not good, good food is not available at your favourite fast-food joint. And then there are some 'I can't . . . I can't stop socializing', 'I had to do some social drinking because my boss or my client was there', 'It's Diwali', 'It's Christmas', 'It's New Year', 'I'll do it from the first week of January', 'Okay, after Easter', 'I have cough and cold', 'My children are too small', 'My children are teen monsters', 'It's my children's carrier time', 'My friends are holding a party', 'I'll look like a fool if I have something healthy'.

Oh, there are so many reasons that 365 days in a year are not enough to lose weight, *but* guess what, you need only one reason to *lose* it. So decide to do it, and read on.

You don't have to rob a bank to get started; you just need to do one small thing at a time.

That little more to reach your weight loss goal may be any of the following:

- starting a walk for ten minutes
- having three to five cups of greens/fruits a day
- doubling your water intake
- fasting once a week
- substituting your fizzy drink with a fresh lime.

You got to be relentless, and you got to be persistent towards the weight loss goal that you want to achieve. And if you want it bad enough, you will make a commitment to fulfil that commitment—keeping up the good work *no matter what*. No matter what it takes, you must keep at it even if it's just a little bit at a time.

First things first, here's a question for you. There are four species on planet Earth who are prone to get fat. Name them in your mind before you see the answer.

- cats
- dogs
- rats
- humans (of course).

This is such a strange question that makes us think, why is it that only us humans and animals under our food guidance (i.e. cats and dogs) are prone to get fat?

Why don't birds get fat? Why not tigers? Why not wolves? Why don't fishes get fat no matter how abundant their food supply from nature?

There is something wrong in the food we eat and not our genes or environmental pollution. Why? Because the same food is making our pet dogs and pet cats fat as well. And we give food to laboratory rats to make them fat as well.

There is something wrong here, fundamentally wrong. Why do almost 70 per cent of humans get fat in the modern world wherever there is abundance of food and only 30 per cent are absolutely healthy despite of these two groups living in the same environment? There are so many whys to wonder about.

The answer might be very simple and complex at the same time.

This book will help you unwind the why and the secret of food, body, psychology, biochemistry, and pathology of obesity.

Having discussed everything in the book, I believe and I know from my personal experience that we become what we think about most of the time. Even if we are genetically prone to get fat, we can change the course of our life if we put our mind and soul in reaching our desired weight.

Chapter 1

This chapter is longer than I thought it would be. Before typing it, before we unfold the secret of nutrition and the calorie puzzle, let me start with the simple fact that your *body* is the most intelligent piece of equipment ever made and it can automatically calculate how much calories it requires to sustain and grow. Now I know you are wondering whether I am right or wrong. Let me make you understand why. There is a regulatory mechanism in your body for everything it is exposed to, be it weather change, food adaptation, physical activity, or any other external variability.

Thermoregulation is the term we use to describe the body's ability to maintain its temperature despite different weather conditions. For example, if the temperature is cold outside, we naturally tend to wear more woollen clothes or multiple layers of clothes, and no one instructs us by calculating external temperature on how many layers we are supposed to wear; it's done by our body naturally without us doing any conscious effort.

Similarly, food intake by our body is regulated naturally through various receptors in our gut, like stretch receptors in the stomach and receptors for macronutrient detection so that certain acids, salts, and enzymes are released by our body to metabolize them, and all these happen automatically without our conscious efforts. We don't need to count calories if the food source is natural and not processed. No other species on earth counts calories; neither should we. It won't be wrong if I say that we are the dumbest species on earth. We count calories to eat, but still 70 per cent of the human population is overweight or obese compared to other species which have no calculations and *no* obesity.

Take physical activity, for example. If we increase aerobic workout, our body adapts naturally by increasing its oxygen-carrying capacity and improving blood circulation in active tissues. All that happens automatically. Increase your weight training, and your body will adapt by increasing muscle size or muscular hypertrophy. Again, it happens on its own.

We humans have somehow started exploiting our body by giving it artificial stimulus in the form of controlled environments, making thermoregulation redundant and in the form of refined foods (sugars and refined cereals), various oils (both saturated and unsaturated), proteins (such as whey, soy, albumin, BCAA or branched-chain amino acid, casein, etc.), making the body's natural feedback mechanism redundant. Then we have exploited physical efforts by following different programs, like pyramid weight training, HITT, circuit training, high-altitude training in artificial oxygen-depleted chambers, and so on. Use of various chemical cocktails like prohormones, EPO, anabolic steroids, growth hormones, insulin, thyroxine, other pharmacological cocktails to increase aerobic capacity, muscle building, muscle stimulation, fat reduction, and so on, making our natural receptors for physical stimulus *redundant*!

To undo all the damage that has occurred to our body, we need to know why we need nutrition. What do various components of food do to our body? And how do we get energy from the food we eat? Let's get started.

Taking up the topic of nutrition and making you understand it is like explaining all the biochemistry and physiology of the body that I studied in medical school and telling you in the context of nutrition what food will have what kind of effect. This chapter will enable you to understand the concept of nutrition just like planet earth, where the blue colour you see is the body of water and the brown-and-green part that you see is the ground on which we humans live.

And though humans are the most intelligent animals on earth, I would hardly be able to mention in a single chapter the information about countries, colour of people, cities, towns, villages, tribes in terms of nutrition, of course. There is a complex process by which living organisms obtain food and use it for growth, metabolism, and repair. So let's start the basics of the journey of food in our body.

The stages of nutrition includes the ingestion of food (what we eat), its digestion, absorption, transport, assimilation, and excretion! No one person can cover diet and nutrition in a single book; it is so vast. That gives me and hundreds of scientists on earth a chance to explore and discover new and innovative ways to improve nutrition, and I believe this will help humankind in pursuit of a better and a healthy life and for you to read as many books as possible on this topic, including the future series of books that I will be writing in my lifetime to help *you*.

The science or study that deals with *food and nourishment* in humans is nutrition. Let's go through some basics of nutrition. Broadly, food is divided into *two* parts—macronutrients and micronutrients.

The macronutrients include:

- carbohydrates
- proteins
- fats.

Carbohydrates

Complex Carbohydrates

As the name suggests, they are complex structures, like our weight loss process is. They are also known as polysaccharides.

Complex carbohydrates have names given by scientists according to the origin, whether carbohydrates are of plant origin and animal origin. We have heard names like *starch* (plant form of carbohydrates) and *glycogen* (polysaccharides or stored carbohydrates in animals, including humans).

Let's take an example by calculating the amount of complex carbohydrates in a human being. Suppose a person is a 70-kilogram female/male; if someone were to calculate the amount of carbohydrates in that person, the results would be as follows:

- The total amount of *blood glucose* would be around 2 to 3 grams (simple carbohydrates).

- The *liver's store* of glycogen would be around 90 grams after a good food intake.
- *Muscles* would have roughly 360 grams of glycogen stored in it.

So the *total amount of glycogen* in that case would be around 450 grams of complex carbohydrates and 2 grams of simple carbohydrates in blood as glucose. Now if we were to calculate the amount of calories stored in the body of that person as carbohydrates, that would be 450 × 4 = 1,800 + 8 kilocalories from simple carbs as 1 gram has 4 calories of energy. So you can assume that the person has roughly 1,800 calories of carbs that are ready to be burned for fuel at any given time. The variation from one person to another will be anywhere between 1,500 to 2,000 calories depending on body composition.

A No-Brainer Tip

If someone says that your blood sugar comes down after an exercise, then you can let them know that it takes at least two to three hours of moderate workout to deplete all glycogen storage in our body. It's only after glycogen depletion that the blood sugar will start going down. If you suffer from hypoglycaemia within one hour of gyming or any kind of workout, please get an appointment with a doctor, you definitely need medical help, not a recovery drink.

Now let's talk about plant-based complex carbs—*starch*. Don't be afraid of this name. It won't make you fat. It's just a name given to hundreds of sugar molecules joined together as a chain known as polysaccharide or starch. This starch is present in all plant-based foods, such as cereals, pulses, beans, vegetables, roots . . . It is virtually in every plant-based food.

There are some *polysaccharides* in plants which cannot be digested by our body, and these are known as non-starch or *fibre*. They include *cellulose*, the most abundant organic molecule on planet earth!

Humans cannot digest cellulose as our genes lack the enzyme to break cellulose into glucose.

The fact that our body cannot digest fibre is the very reason we should have at least some of it in our diet. We should have at least 25 grams of fibre in our total diet every day to add bulk to the stools and prevent that aching constipation, so please add them to your daily quota.

There are two types of fibre in our food—*soluble* and *insoluble* fibre. Both are needed for proper functioning of the digestive system. In case you are constipated even if you take sufficient amount of fibre in your diet, you need to meet your doctor to have your metabolic diagnosis done or to rule out any other underlying pathology.

Vegetarians don't have to take any extra fibre; if you mainly have plant-based food, your fibre intake is sufficient almost by default. Just to give you an example, one bowl of cooked beans have roughly 20 grams of fibre—practically all your daily need. Our body doesn't need much of anything. Probably, it's overnutrition that's killing us—or is there something more complex than that!

Simple Carbohydrates

I deliberately forgot to put some light on simple carbs before complex carbs.

In chemistry terms, simple carbohydrates are also known as *monosaccharides* and disaccharides. Or we should say that simple carbohydrates are the backbone of the food-processing industry and all the sweets in the world have simple carbs. Greeks gave it the suffix *-ose* at the end of its names—glucose, fructose, galactose, sucrose, lactose, maltose, etc.

In the modern world, we know these carbohydrates by names such as fructose corn syrup, fudge filling, dextrose, cracker meal, corn starch, brown sugar, molasses, caramel, and many more!

A No-Brainer Tip

If you give your body a lot of simple carbohydrates, especially man-made carbohydrates, you are not using the full potential of all the complex chemical reactions that should happen in your body to extract glucose and energy. Your body has all the ways and means to convert starch (complex carbs) in food into glucose, which is taken up by the blood and used by every cell in your body in forming energy or ATP (adenosine triphosphate), the energy power source of the body.

Just to give you a brief introduction to what happens when you eat your carbohydrates and how you get that energy from them, let's skim through this mysterious world of carbohydrate digestion, and if you want vivid details, I recommend you join a medical school. LOL.

Starch------glucose------energy (ATP)

Some excess of starch is stored as glycogen in the muscles and liver. And if some more glucose is left, it is converted into fat store for later use.

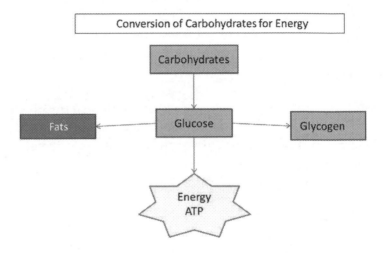

The *ticket* for *blood glucose* to enter the body cells is *insulin*. The more glucose in the blood, the more insulin (tickets) will be released to regulate the blood sugar and avail it for energy and storage. Interestingly, insulin is a *universal ticket* for not only glucose *but* also for fats. These too are transported into fat cells with the help of insulin. *More insulin* means *more fat from blood* into fat cells, and your fat cells grow happily ever after. Again this is an oversimplification of a very complex process happening in the body.

If it were that simple, I would have stopped here, *but* there is a twist in the story of carbohydrates. A lot of *carbohydrates* are physiologically different. It is getting complicated, I know, but you know, so is life. Throughout their lives, people such as doctors, registered dieticians, food engineers, or biochemists try to perfect these details, just like a geologist who works to study the earth, master in business administration who manages your business, and so on. So bear with me for some time. If you don't have medical background, you will find it a bit difficult when you first read it, and then you will get the hang of it.

Digestion and *absorption* of carbohydrates are different for every food item, and we scientists have given it a unique name: GI. GI, or glycaemic index, is the rate at which any food item increases blood sugar levels after we ingest it.

Glucose is taken as the standard around which all other carbohydrates are compared. The GI of glucose is taken as 100.

Let's say, for example, that we take an *apple*. Apple has a GI of 34, which means that if you consume 50 grams of apple, your blood glucose concentration will rise to the level that reaches 34 per cent in comparison to the blood sugar rise with 50 grams of glucose.

The glycaemic index range of various food items are mentioned as follows:

Vegetables

Low GI	Glycemic Index
Green Peas	39
Sweet Corn (frozen)	47
Raw Carrots	16
Boiled Carrots	41
Eggplant/Aubergine	15
Broccoli	10
Cauliflower	15
Cabbage	10
Mushrooms	10
Tomatoes	15
Chillies	10
Lettuce	10
Green Beans	15
Red Peppers	10
Onions	10

Medium GI

Beetroot	64

High GI

Pumpkin	75
Parsnips	97

Dairy

Low GI	Glycemic Index
Whole milk	31
Skimmed milk	32
Chocolate milk	42
Sweetened yoghurt	33
Artificially Sweetened Yoghurt	23
Custard	35
Soy Milk	44

Medium GI

Ice cream	63

Legumes (Beans)

Low GI	Glycemic index
Kidney Beans (canned)	52
Butter Beans	36
Chick Peas	42
Haricot/Navy Beans	31
Lentils, Red	21
Lentils, Green	30
Pinto Beans	45
Blackeyed Beans	50
Yellow Split Peas	32
Medium GI	
Beans in Tomato Sauce	56

Breads

Low GI	Glycemic Index
Soya and Linseed	36
Wholegrain Pumpernickel	46
Heavy Mixed Grain	45
Whole Wheat	49
Sourdough Rye	48
Sourdough Wheat	54
Medium GI	
Croissant	67
Hamburger bun	61
Pita, white	57
Whole meal Rye	62

Other Common foods

Low GI	Glycemic Index
Wheat Pasta	54
New Potatoes	54
Meat Ravioli	39
Spaghetti	32
Tortellini (Cheese)	50
Egg Fettuccini	32
Brown Rice	50
Buckwheat	51
White long grain rice	50
Pearled Barley	22
Yam	35
Sweet Potatoes	48
Instant Noodles	47
Wheat tortilla	30

Medium GI	
Basmati Rice	58
Couscous	61
Cornmeal	68
Taco Shells	68
Gnocchi	68
Canned Potatoes	61
Chinese (Rice) Vermicelli	58
Baked Potatoes	60
Wild Rice	57

High GI	
Instant White Rice	87
Glutinous Rice	86
Short Grain White Rice	83
Tapioca	70
Fresh Mashed Potatoes	73
French Fries	75
Instant Mashed Potatoes	80

Breakfast Cereals

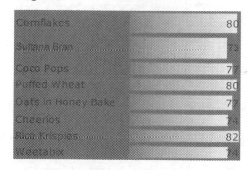

Low GI

	Glycemic Index	
All-bran		50
Oat bran		50
Rolled Oats		51
Special K meals		54
Natural Muesli		40
Porridge		52

Medium GI

Bran Buds		58
Mini Wheat		58
Nutrigrain		66
Shredded Wheat		67
Porridge Oats		63

High GI

Cornflakes		80
Sultana Bran		73
Coco Pops		77
Puffed Wheat		80
Oats in Honey Bake		77
Cheerios		74
Rice Krispies		82
Weetabix		74

The higher the GI value, the higher the rise of blood sugar and the more insulin released by the body to regulate it, and as we have mentioned earlier, increase in insulin will deposit more fat in fat tissues. Therefore, foods with higher GI values are more fattening.

Note: In medical conditions, if your body cannot release a sufficient amount of insulin (or the body is resistant to insulin functions), then there is a rise in blood sugar with intake of food. This is known as diabetes mellitus type 2, which is a metabolic disease of carbohydrate metabolism.

Proteins

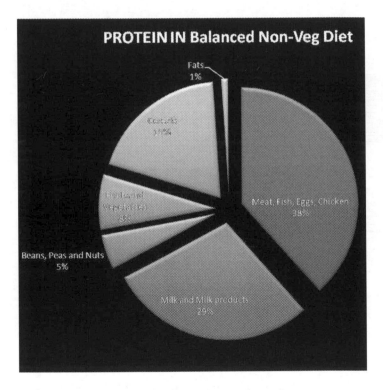

The only difference between this *macronutrient* and carbohydrates is that protein *has nitrogen* apart from carbon, oxygen, and hydrogen present in the other two macronutrients (fats and carbohydrates). There are some proteins that can be associated with other elements— like *iron* (haemoglobin), phosphorus, *sulphur*, cobalt— depending upon various functions of the body.

Again, a 70-kilogram adult like me will have between *9 to 11 kilograms* of protein in my body. Just like glycogen, which is a chain of glucose molecules, protein is a chain of *amino acids*. There are more than *fifty* amino acids in our body. In fact, our body has more than 50,000 protein-containing compounds made with combinations of these amino acids.

Now these amino acids are of *two* known types.

1. *Essential amino acids*, as the name suggests, cannot be synthesized in our body at a good rate and have to come from our diet; they are essential amino acids. There are eight essential amino acids in adults, and in infants, there are nine of them. *Histidine* is an essential amino acid in infants, but our body starts synthesizing it later in life. The remaining *eight* amino acids we've got to get from our diet are as follows: *valine*, leucine, *lysine*, isoleucine, *methionine*, phenylalanine, *threonine*, and tryptophan.
2. The other twelve amino acids are *non-essential because* they are made in our body using compounds already existing in the body to meet the demands for growth development and for wear and tear of muscles during exercise.

Proteins consist of around 15 per cent of the body weight. Again, I am doing oversimplification of facts which are complex. The protein concentrations of different cells are different. For example, in the *brain*, protein content is not more than *10 per cent*, and on the other hand, the RBC and muscles have almost *20 per cent* protein in their basic composition.

- *Structural proteins* **are found in** hair, *nails*, bones, *tendons*, muscles, *ligaments*, etc.
- Globular proteins make more than 1,500 enzymes that take part in *regulating the metabolism* of carbohydrates, proteins, and fats for energy production.

A No-Brainer Tip

Non-vegetarians don't have to worry about their protein intake because there is always a sufficient amount of amino-acid reserves in non-vegetarian diet. The main concern of inadequacy of this macronutrient is in the *vegan* group of people. Vegans are purely on plants and supplements. Vegans should have *more grains* and *pulses* with nuts to compensate essential protein lack. Lacto-vegetarians (people who consume dairy products) and lacto-ovo-vegetarians (vegetarians who consume eggs and dairy products) have sufficient amounts of amino-acid pool and never get protein malnutrition.

A Myth Worth Busting

Muscle mass doesn't increase by eating a high-protein diet. If extra protein was the only reason behind gain in muscle mass, eating 100 grams of extra protein over and above the daily recommended allowance would had converted it into muscle, and everyone would be supermen and superwomen, but this extra protein is deaminated and stored as *body fat*!

One of the main reasons gymgoers don't lose weight is the fact that they take too much protein in the form of whey protein powders, thinking that it will repair micro tears after exercise. Yes, you definitely need extra protein as supplementation, provided you are working out more than five hours every day, like athletes do. A person who does just one to two hours of workout won't require protein. A balanced diet gives you sufficient proteins for muscle repair.

The reason we sports doctors give protein supplements to the athletes is because they do four to seven hours of vigorous exercises. Prolonged exercise redistributes blood to the muscular system to keep supplying oxygen and nutrients to them, and that causes lack of blood supply to the digestive system in an athlete. Just imagine that when you have 5 litres of blood in your body and most of the blood is pooled to the muscle tissues for three hours in the morning and then again for around three hours in the evening trainings, would your digestive system get enough blood supply to properly absorb even macronutrients like protein and carbohydrates?

So if you want to *lose weight*, it's my belief that you should not to look at protein supplements unless you are replacing your major meal for a protein shake. The point to be noted is that if your workouts are more than three hours a day, carbohydrate and protein supplements should be seriously considered for recovery.

Fats

Fats present in our body are known as *lipids*, which consist mainly of carbon and hydrogen with a dash of oxygen. Storage of fat happens in *fat cells* or *adipocytes*. *Interestingly*, evolution has always favoured the idea of stored fat! It's because stored fat is meant for emergencies when there is no food or less food.

The question is, where is that emergency now? Thanks to great storage techniques and refrigerators, we have abundant food all around for us, don't we? Maybe you are storing that excess fat for World War III. That's when we will have short supply of food, and only people who have extra layers of fat will survive—the optimistic side for gaining fat mass!

Normally, the fat content of the human body is and should be between 16 to 30 per cent.

In our body, fats are present as *eicosanoids* and *fatty acids*.

- Fatty acids—these can be *saturated* fatty acids, which has a single bond on all carbon atoms, or unsaturated fatty acids, which are mono- and polyunsaturated fatty acids, which means one or more than one double bonds in carbon atoms are present.
- Steroids—these are all made up of *four* interconnected *rings of carbon atoms* with a *hydroxyl* group attached to it. Examples of steroids naturally found in the body are *cholesterol*, cortisol, oestrogen (female sex hormone), and testosterone (male sex hormone). Oestrogen is made from fat cells in both males and females. Excess of body fat

increases oestrogen, which can even cause *cancer*. Testosterone is also present in females, where they are known as *androgens*.

- Triglycerides—this is the molecule we commonly refer to as fat, sometimes *bad fat*. It is formed from glycerol (an alcohol) plus *three fatty acids*. These two combine in a chemical reaction with the removal of water to form triglycerides.

On the other hand, the breakdown of fats *requires water* for production of fatty acids and glycerol to release *energy, as shown below*.

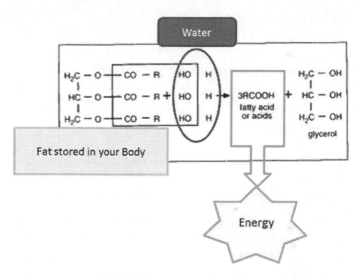

That's why your doctors, dieticians, and fitness trainers tell you to hydrate yourself. It actually helps *burn fat*!

The following are the functions of fat in our body:

- Fat acts as an energy reserve. We all have it plenty around our waist though.☺

- Fat helps transport fat-soluble vitamins (I discuss this later in this chapter).
- Fat helps in hormone production.
- Fat protects our vital organs.

So there is a minimum fat percentage that we need to have in our body, which is essential to maintain the smooth running of body functions.

There are critical levels of fat percentage below which the essential functions of fats will be hampered, and those should be above

- ➢ 4 per cent for males
- ➢ 12 per cent for females.

In Indian females, my practical experience shows that menstrual disturbances start at around 16 per cent or below, and in Indian males, hormonal imbalance starts below 6 per cent.

Now let's do some *calculation*s. I am 70 kilograms in weight and my *fat percentage is 16*. So the fat stored in my body should be around 11.2 kilograms of pure, unadulterated fat. Now if we calculate the energy stored in that 11.2 kilograms of fat (as we all know, 1 gram of fat releases 9 calories of energy), so the number of calories I can get from my fat storage is *100,800 calories*! That's sufficient for a year of my exercise without consuming a drop of oil! I am doing oversimplification again, but that gives you an idea of the enormous amount of energy stored in just 11.2 kilograms of fat.

A No-Brainer Tip

Our body doesn't start utilizing fat right from the start of the exercise. Scientists experimented and found that if you continue exercising for more than three hours at a stretch, 50 to 60 per cent of energy will come from your body's stored fat. And before that, during the first hour of exercise, the percentage of fat burned by our body is around 10 to 20 per cent of the total energy consumed.

Excess of Fats, Proteins, and Carbohydrates Can Cause Weight Gain!

I don't know whether you know this *fact*, but *all* the main macronutrients (namely *carbohydrates*, *fats*, and *proteins*) can all convert into one another in the human body, and all can provide energy when needed!

Let's do a superfast brush-up and eyeball the idea of how all three macronutrients (fats, proteins, and carbs) can provide energy and how glucose forms protein, protein forms glucose, glucose forms fat, and protein forms fat! It is a fascinating world in our body. As we've read earlier, all macronutrients are formed of carbon, hydrogen, oxygen, and nitrogen, so why can't our body add nitrogen to carbohydrates to form proteins or remove nitrogen and most of oxygen to form fats? Guess what, it *does* and does them well. How is it possible?

After a super crash course on our three main macronutrients, let's find out how all three of them form *ATP*, the energy source of our body and the fuel for metabolism.

All three macronutrients can enter the Krebs cycle (it's just another name given to the sequence of steps for energy production which helps using food in our body for energy formation).

In the diagram, you can see that there are three steps in the energy cycle. *Pyruvate*, *oxaloacetate*, and acetyl CoA are common in glucose and protein metabolism, so they can interchange among themselves and back and forth into fat and energy. Even the *glycerol* portion of fat can be converted back into glucose. As you can see in the diagram below, fatty acids can be used to synthesize keto acids, which help form amino acids and hence into proteins. So our metabolism is a complex biochemical reaction, a porridge of processes in which everything is related to everything else.

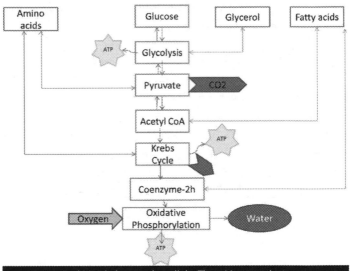

Fuel Metabolism Involves all the Three Macronutrients

So the names *fat*, *protein*, and *carbohydrate* are to make us understand the differences between them, but for our body, they are not very different. All of them can be used as energy sources if blood glucose is lacking. Each of the macronutrients can provide the raw material required to make the most of other two macronutrients. That's why we doctors say anything in excess will be converted into fat. Be it excess carbohydrates, excess fats, or even excess proteins—these will all be converted into fat.

So the total number of calories always matter. Again, it is more complex than you think. I mean, who says losing weight is easy? It indeed is *rocket science*, especially for those of you who can't lose weight despite all your efforts!

Micronutrients

These are substances, such as *vitamins* and *trace elements*, essential for healthy growth, repair, facilitation of energy flow and transfer, tissue synthesis, and development of our body, but they are required in very small amounts, hence micronutrients.

Your doctor might need some battery of tests to determine deficiency of micronutrients in your present diet because *everyone has* different rate-limiting steps depending on their gene coding and millions of reactions taking place in the body.

Sometimes we prescribe extra micronutrient intake, and the length of time for which the prescription is required may vary from five days to three months depending on:

- the condition of health
- the illness, which can cause deficiencies in the organ system of the body that is affected
- possible genetic deficiencies in a particular biochemical reaction
- some external conditions, like extreme stress, that can cause deficiencies
- deficiencies that may be caused by our diet.

A Myth Worth Busting

It will be so dumb to say that nowadays the nutrients in food are depleted so everybody must pop in a multivitamin pill to cover the deficiencies. I could have increased the sales of this book by mentioning that you should take this or that exotic miracle pill that will do this to you. It would have increased the curiosity. Or if some pharmaceutical company had sponsored me, I would have promoted them as well.

But I have to tell you the truth, and the truth is that 40 per cent of the world's population still doesn't pop in any multivitamin or mineral pills and still live a normal life. I'll surely discuss multivitamins and minerals in detail in some of my future books, but right now, it is beyond the scope of this book for me to go in depth into it, though we will skim through.

Blast from the Past

I was a team doctor for Indian Athletics for more than two years. In that tenure, I came across almost 3,000 players from various schemes like the national camp, Commonwealth camp, Olympic camp, Sports Authority of India's Training Centres Scheme (STC) for boys and girls, and various regional and zonal camps. I had been with the best of the best athletes, and you will be surprised that almost 65 per cent of them were from very poor backgrounds and couldn't afford to buy supplements while training for six hours a day!

Once, I remember, six years back, the team coach of senior women for the 400 metres came to me to discuss supplements schedule for the players. 'I am talking about those girl athletes who had won gold in Commonwealth 2010.' When this coach asked me for help, in the next three days, I saw and analysed their biochemistry test results and training phase (it was the pre-competition phase, one of the hardest phases of training). We prepared a list of supplements to be given to the girls, and I handed that list to the coach. After two days, the coach came back to me with a complaint and said, 'The supplements cost INR 25,000 for each girl, and they can't afford them.' That day, I realized that a lot of players were doing sports without the help of any supplements and even without multivitamins just because they couldn't afford it. Whatever they earned from their government job and their prize money from competition wins, they would send it home. Most of them had camp food and nothing else. Many of them had achieved their goals and had made their nation proud in various international competitions.

That was the moment I realized that humans have immense power within us. My practical experience shows that a lot of multivitamins work as placebo. The food that is produced from the earth (non-genetic-engineered and non-processed food) is not lacking in micronutrients in any way. Your body might be lacking in certain enzymes which may prevent you from absorbing some minerals, and for that, we can always do detailed biochemistry tests to find out. I am sure your weight loss experts and doctors will get your detailed tests done before enrolling you into any weight loss programs.

Homework

I highly recommend that you know which specific vitamin, mineral, or hormone you are lacking and what kind of supplements you need and for how many days or months you should be taking those supplements under the guidance of your family doctor; this would be a good idea.

Let's briefly discuss the *micronutrients* that are required by our body. Why do we need them? What are their role in keeping our body healthy?

Vitamins

The word *vitamin* was coined in 1911 by biochemist Casimir Funk because it was discovered and believed that the chemical was necessary to life and it was a chemical amine. And later when this group evolved, scientists knew that not all vitamins were always amines so letter e in the end was later removed. Its original name was *vit-amine*.

The *two* broad classifications of vitamins are:

- fat-soluble vitamins (A, D, E, and K)

  In our body, vitamins A, D, and K are stored in the liver, and vitamin E is distributed in all fatty tissues.

Symptoms of fat-soluble-vitamin deficiency may not appear for years because they can be stored in your body for future use for a long time.

- water-soluble vitamins

  All B vitamins and vitamin C are water-soluble vitamins and are safe to have without prescription because any excess will be excreted within twenty-four hours. These vitamins are required by our body every day, and so our food should be rich in these vitamins.

Note: There is no difference between natural and artificial vitamins. Some manufacturers have this strategy to advertise vitamins as natural. They are just chemicals with a specific chemical formula; some are better absorbed than others. Whether made in a laboratory or in nature, they are the same chemicals. Water will always be H_2O regardless of being mineral or tap or organic water; it will still be H_2O.

See the table for details on vitamins.

Vitamin	Where is it from? (Food source)	Uses in our body	Recommended dietary allowance for adults	Deficiency disease	Upper intake level	Overdose danger
vitamin A (retinol, carotenoids)	green vegetables, all red fruits and vegetables (pumpkin, tomato, papaya, peach, apricot, carrots) chicken liver, egg yolks, milk cheese, fortified margarine	making of visual pigments; growth and repair of skin, bones, teeth, and connective tissues; a potent antioxidant	900 µg	night blindness, permanent blindness, loss of appetite, acne, skin disease and dryness, hyperkeratosis, and keratomalacia	3,000 µg	vomiting, skin pealing, swelling of bones, hypervitaminosis A
vitamin B₁ (thiamine)	all whole cereals (they have B₁ in abundance), legumes, liver, pork	digestion of carbohydrates (nature has it all), with carbohydrates cereals give us B₁ to digest starch (a good reason to have whole grains), reduction of mental clouding	1.2 mg	beriberi, depression, poor memory, *fatigue*, Wernicke–Korsakoff syndrome	not specified	drowsiness or muscle relaxation with large doses

vitamin B$_2$ (riboflavin)	*yogurt*, cheese, chicken liver, fish, *spinach*, all green vegetables (it's quite abundant in your food and relatively heat-stable)	formation of FAD and FMN required for steps in energy production	1.3 mg	eye lesions, ariboflavinosis, constipation, diarrhoea, cheilosis	not set	not detected
vitamin B$_3$ (niacin)	all whole grains (including brown rice), lean meat, egg yolk, dairy products	formation of NAD+ and NADP, required practically in all *oxidation-reduction reactions* in the body	16 mg	*fatigue*, pellagra, reduced sexual functions, lack of motivation	35 mg	liver damage, flushing, burning and tingling in whole body
vitamin B$_5$ (pantothenic acid)	whole wheat, rye, barley, nut, green leafy vegetables, egg yolk, chicken	metabolism of fats and carbohydrates, basically for energy metabolism and immunity	5 mg	paresthesia, depression, adrenal fatigue, *respiratory infections*	No limit	diarrhoea, nausea, and heartburn
vitamin B$_6$ (pyridoxine)	*wheat germ* (this is rich in B$_6$), green vegetables, chicken, egg yolk, all meats	*body healing and repair*, protein and glycogen metabolism, mood regulations	1.5 mg	PMS, depression, dandruff, asthma, anaemia, peripheral neuropathy	100 mg	impairment of proprioception, nerve damage (doses >100 mg/day)

biotin	brown rice, fruits, legumes, *yeast*, chicken liver, egg yolk	glycogen formation, *metabolism* of proteins and fats	30 µg	*fatigue*, nausea, dermatitis, enteritis	not specified	not reported
vitamin B_9 (folic acid)	carrots, whole wheat, rye, pumpkin, green vegetables, avocados	building the body's defence, carbohydrate and protein metabolism	400 µg	megaloblast but no anaemia, red tongue, *diarrhoea*, and neural tube defects (deficiency of this vitamin during pregnancy is associated *with birth defects*)	1,000 µg	may mask symptoms of vitamin B_{12} deficiency
vitamin B_{12} (cyanocobalamin)	red meat, chicken, shellfish, dairy products, blue-green algae (in fact, it is the only plant source, so pure vegans should take it as supplement)	growth, healing, and repair of body tissues; production of red blood cells; and neural functions	2.4 µg	*fatigue*, neurological disorders, *anaemia*	not specified	acne-like rashes

vitamin C (ascorbic acid)	kiwi, guava, all citrus fruits, watermelon, strawberries, pepper, cabbage, spinach, broccoli, tomato, green salads	immunity, health and repair of gums and skin, wound healing	100 mg	pcor wound healing, *frequent infections,* scurvy	2,000 mg	beyond 2 g, it is found to cause kidney stones
vitamin D	dairy products, cod liver oil, fish, egg yolk, sunlight (made in the body with *sunlight,* one hour of basking in sunlight for our daily dose)	health of bones and teeth, increase in calcium absorption, promotion of growth, mood elevation	10 µg	rickets, non-alignment of teeth, *muscular weakness,* osteomalacia	50 µg	hypervitaminosis D, kidney damage, weight loss, vomiting, diarrhoea
vitamin E (tocopherol)	whole grains (especially the germ part of grain), egg yolk, oily fishes, soy beans, seeds, margarines, nuts	immunity booster, skin health, a strong antioxidant, improvement of wound healing	15 mg	deficiency is very rare, and patient may complain *of flaky skin,* palpitation, *anæmia,* even mild haemolytic anæmia in newborn infants	1,000 mg	increased chances of CHF (congestive heart failure)

vitamin K (phylloquinone)	yogurt, green leafy vegetables, fruits, egg yolk, fish oil, and meat	blood clot factor, bone repair and building	120 µg	osteoporosis, *bleeding diathesis*, including heavy menstrual flow and easy bruising	no maximum limit	increased coagulation and liver damage

Minerals

Approximately *4 per cent* of our body is minerals. Minerals are divided into *two main* categories depending upon the body requirement.

- Minerals that are required more than 100 milligrams per twenty-four hours are classified as *major minerals*
- Those which are required in lesser quantity are known as *trace minerals*.

Just go through the table below to know the details of these minerals.

Dietary mineral	Quantity needed	Foods rich in specific mineral	Recommended for adults	Major functions in the body	Deficiency	Excess
calcium	major	dairy products, fish, soybeans, dried legumes, almonds, dark-green vegetables	1,300 mg	proper functioning of muscles, heart and digestive system health, building of bone mass, blood clot, and nerve transmission	stunted growth, hypocalcaemia, *rickets*, convulsions	hypercalcaemia, including fatigue, anorexia, nausea, vomiting, pancreatitis, and increased urination
sodium	major	table salt, milk, even vegetables like spinach	1,500 mg	acid–base balance, a systemic electrolyte, essential in co-regulating ATP with potassium, nerve function	muscle cramps, *weakness*, hyponatremia	hypernatremia, high blood pressure
chlorine, chloride	major	table salt, some vegetables and fruits	2,300 mg	important part of extracellular fluid, needed for production of hydrochloric acid in the stomach and in cellular pump functions	very rare to cause hypochloraemia	contributing factor to increased blood pressure, hyperchloraemia

magnesium	major	whole grains, green leafy vegetables, citrus fruits, almonds, mushrooms, sweetcorn, onion, garlic, figs, carrots, resins, soybeans, even dairy products	420 mg	activation of protein synthesis, heart health, mental clarity, processing of ATP, and bone health	muscle cramps, spasm, behavioural disturbances, *growth failure*, hypomagnesaemia	diarrhoea, hypermagnesaemia
potassium	major	potato, banana, almonds, milk, meat, lima beans, cantaloupe, spinach, asparagus, figs, peanuts, sesame seeds	4,700 mg	nerve transmission, acid–base balance, important electrolyte, essential in forming ATP with sodium	muscle cramps, frequent thirst, tingling in extremities, mental confusion, *loss of appetite*, hypokalaemia	hyperkalemia if kidney function is not good, cardiac arrhythmia
phosphorus	major	milk and milk products, meat, poultry, fish, whole grains	700 mg	an important component of bone cells and teeth formation, energy processing, and acid–base balance of the body	demineralization of bones, loss of calcium, *weakness*, hypophosphatemia	hyperphosphatemia and erosion of jaw

Mineral		Sources	RDA	Function	Deficiency symptoms	Excess symptoms
zinc	trace	chicken liver, shellfish, turkey, brown rice, pumpkin, cashews, all whole grains, chickpeas, tofu, soybeans	11 mg	protein metabolism, immunity, required for proper functioning of so many enzymes (such as carboxypeptidase, liver alcohol dehydrogenase, and carbonic anhydrase), sperm formation, wound healing	small sex glands, *poor wound healing*, growth retardation, *frequent infections*, excessive PMS, flecks on fingernails	fever, nausea, vomiting, diarrhoea
iodine	trace	seafood, dairy products, blue-green algae, iodized salt, garlic, and other vegetables	150 µg	synthesis of thyroid hormones, thyroxine, and triiodothyronine; prevention of goitre; immune system booster	*goitre*, weight gain, reduced energy, constipation, cold extremities, reduced sweating	high intake of iodine suppresses thyroid activity
iron	trace	red meat, eggs, dark-green vegetables, fish, dry fruits, whole grains, legumes, and fortified cereals	18 mg	required for many proteins and enzymes, important structure of haemoglobin, maintaining bone structure, growth of overall body structure	*anaemia, weakness,* infections, brittle nails, depression	haemochromatosis, cirrhosis of liver

manganese	trace	rye, oats, brown rice, walnuts, hazelnuts, lentils	2.3 mg	cofactor in enzyme function, blood sugar control, bone repair, antioxidant, nerve tissue maintenance	dizziness, irritability, *general fatigue,* and reduced fertility in females	manganism and fatty liver
selenium	trace	meat, all seafood, grains, sesame seeds, lentils, beans, sea fish, chicken liver, sunflower seeds	55 µg	a cofactor essential for activity of antioxidant enzymes, **immune system booster,** heart protective, and live detoxification, its function closely resembles that of vitamin E	frequent infections, *poor wound healing,* signs of ageing, chronic fatigue, anaemia	gastrointestinal disorder, lung irritation
copper	trace	meat, drinking water kept in a copper vessel	900 µg	component of many redox enzymes, including cytochrome c oxidase and other enzyme action in digestive system	*bone changes,* anaemia (rare)	copper toxicity, as in Wilson's disease

Now we have gone through minerals, and you might have noticed that the main roles that they play in humans are the following:

1. helps in the *functioning* of heart rhythm, muscle contraction, nerve conduction, and acid–base balance
2. provides *structure* to the body by being part of the bones, teeth, and RBC in blood
3. helps in anabolism and catabolism of macronutrients, thus *maintaining* a balanced body.

Let's simplify the contribution of some minerals to *anabolism* (picture 1) and *catabolism* (in picture 2) of macronutrients in a diagrammatical way:

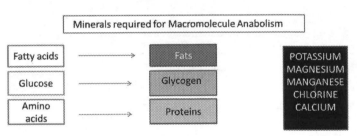

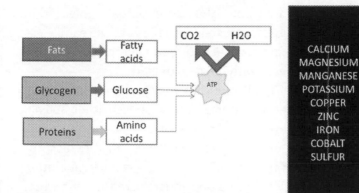

Water

The discussion about food and nutrition is incomplete without water (or should I say *divine water*), without which life on earth wouldn't have existed in the first place. We had a wonderful blog which I had written about water. It sums up the importance of water in our body.

> Everyone knows that we need at least two litres of water every day to keep our body healthy and for that great-looking skin.

> I must refresh your memory of its importance and the magic that water does in your body and why we health experts keep on encouraging you to stay hydrated; some of the functions will sound familiar to you.

This is what I have to say about this holy liquid:

- Water transports the nutrients that you eat from your digestive system into the bloodstream.
- Waste products of your body in the form of urine and faeces with the help of water.
- Watery fluids lubricate your joints, keeping bony surfaces from grinding against each other, and no, it's not the oil as I hear a lot of my patients saying.
- Water, due to its heat-stabilizing qualities, absorbs a lot of heat, maintaining a constant temperature in your body, so you must increase your water intake in extreme heat and cold.
- Water provides transport and is a medium for all metabolic reactions, and thus, it increases your metabolism and helps you lose some weight, making you look good.
- Water cannot be compressed, and it is 60 to 70 per cent of your body, providing volume and form to the body. Without water, your body is just 30 per cent!

And do we all know what is left after all the water evaporates in the cremation furnace?

You guys are intelligent enough to answer that.

Drink some to lose some fat. I am talking about water, people!

Stay hydrated, and stay healthy. ☺ (From my blog archive)

Always ask your doctor before starting any micronutrient supplementation, especially if you are suffering from some chronic disease. And don't worry, doctors will always prescribe you the micronutrients that are best suited for your condition and not what are suggested by quacks as they can have detrimental effects on health, even life-threatening conditions. In case you have forgotten the overdose effects of vitamins and minerals in the table, read again.

Summary

- Your food has two main nutrients: macronutrients and micronutrients.
- The macronutrients in your diet are made of carbon, hydrogen, oxygen, and nitrogen as the primary elements in them, and these macronutrients are proteins, carbohydrates, and fats.
- The combination of oxygen, carbon, and hydrogen in a specific manner forms carbohydrates and fats. Proteins have majorly one extra element (i.e. nitrogen) along with the other three elements.
- Calorie distribution in typical diets all over the world is 50 per cent carbohydrates, 30 per cent fats, and 20 per cent proteins.
- Our body has a unique capacity to produce energy from any of these macromolecules, and excess of any of the three will inevitably increase body fat.
- Micronutrients in a diet help in energy transfer and synthesis of tissues.
- The two micronutrients are vitamins and minerals.

- There are thirteen known vitamins; of them, four are the fat-soluble vitamins A, D, E, and K and the water-soluble vitamins (B group of vitamins) and vitamin C.
- The other group of micronutrients is minerals. Minerals are everywhere in nature (in water, in soil, everywhere), and our body has 4 per cent minerals by weight.
- Minerals are an important part of enzymes and provide structure to bones, teeth, and metabolic reactions of macronutrients.
- And do consider water as an important nutrient, without which we can't survive a day.

Chapter 2

Why Is Weight Loss a Losing Battle for So Many of Us?

Overweight or obesity, what exactly is this battleground? What is this ghost we all are fighting against?

When weight loss experts throughout the world say that everything is as simple as 'eat less, move your body, and lose weight', why is this simple formula of energy in versus energy out effective only in a few cases and very ineffective in a majority of obese or overweight people?

Let's try unravel this mystical world of weight loss.

To lose 10 kilograms of weight and 4 inches from my problem area for aesthetic reasons to feel good and confident—that was what I wanted in my early twenties, and I struggled hard to show my six-pack and be a successful model and bodybuilder back in my college days. And then on the other side, there were people around me who needed to lose 20, 40, or even 100 kilograms of those extra layers of fat for medical reasons to live a disease-free and comfortable life.

For me, losing weight was a real effort, and in my journey to good health of over twenty years, I saw that for some folks out there, losing weight was as easy as playing a game. And then there were some people who lost weight very quickly at a young age, and then suddenly somehow, the body stopped responding no matter what diet they followed to lose that fat stored in their bodies. In some people, nothing worked no matter what; it became a struggle for life. It was a losing battle! Why? Because weight loss is a rocket science and we have to dig deep for answers!

As you all know, WHO (World Health Organization) has declared obesity as a chronic disease and a global threat to health. In other words, being overweight is the recipe for disaster. Sadly, everyone who is obese was once mildly overweight. So a good advice would be to try to stabilize your weight at pre-risk levels or take expert advice to keep your weight down for your health.

It is easier to gain weight than to lose weight, but it is not tough to maintain good health. 'Yes, we know all that, but it's getting tough to maintain good health, isn't it?'

In my early years of weight loss practice, my knowledge about weight loss was no more than skin-deep (calorie in versus calorie out). My sister has been working with me through all these years of our search for alchemy in this field, and we found some interesting facts along the way to good health which I would like to share with you in this chapter and the following chapters to make what is unknown known—of course, starting with what is known.

> A lot of people come to us and don't agree on reducing their fat and refined-sugar intake, saying, 'These are things we have been eating for generations.' Well, I thought, Let's dig

out some data on how our current diets are different from past generations. Here's what I found. It will surprise you.

As human beings, we are made up of approximately two-thirds water, one-fourth protein, and the rest is fat and a few minerals and vitamins. Every single molecule comes from what we eat and drink. Eating the highest-quality food in right quantities helps you to achieve your highest potential for health.

Modern diets have drifted far from the ideal intake in the past trends. The pie charts below show what we are eating right now in comparison to previous generations. In the last century, particularly the last three decades, we have started eating too much fat, refined carbohydrates, salt, and too less fibre.

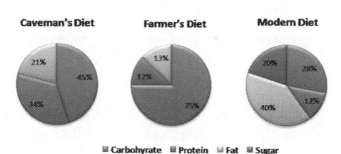

Part of the problem of increased obesity is the modern lifestyle. As our lives speed up, we spend less time cooking and become more reliant on processed food. I have been on the other side of the table; when our team worked on developing new processed foods, our focus was always to make food which was tasty and had a long shelf life. Nutrition was never on the cards, and that's what processed-food philosophy is.

So if you plan to lose some weight, you can only do one thing. Go back to the diet our earlier generations were eating (some 70– 100 years back). (Nidhi Mohan Kamal, weight loss consultant, www.nidsun.org

Sometimes I get frustrated at the recovery pace of some of my patients. Out of the 4,100 patients we have treated till I wrote this book, 100 of them were virtually unaffected by all our best efforts put together. These were the clients who made us realize that we had to learn much more than we knew about the science of weight loss and implemented it and that we needed to sharpen our skills and knowledge and evolve ourselves to help them.

Some questions haunt every scientist and every healthcare provider in the world, questions like 'Why is it that more than 50 per cent of the population have become overweight in the past twenty years?', 'Why is it that we and thousands of researchers all over the world have not been able to decode the mystery of weight gain?', and 'Is there a single solution to this epidemic?'

Let's simplify what *obesity* means and what is already well *known*.

Obesity means there is an excess of body fat (more than the normal amount of stored fat in fat cells). It is associated with at least two of the following things:

- glucose intolerance
- insulin resistance
- diabetes type 2
- dyslipidemia (increased triglycerides, LDL, and decreased HDL)
- hypertension
- cancer
- tummy fat or omental fat or visceral fat
- increased risk of heart disease
- osteoarthritis
- lower-back pain
- elevated C-reactive protein
- depression
- lack of energy
- PCOD
- hypothyroidism.

VAT (visceral adipose tissue) is the most dangerous type of fat.

It's not the total weight of the body but the *weight* contributed by fat in your body that is responsible for the risk of all medical conditions. For medical reasons, the most dangerous fat is that in your tummy.

How to Know That My Extra Weight Is Due to Fat and Not to Bones or Muscles

The easy *test for detection* for being overweight is by measuring a person's waist circumference. Even this test is an oversimplification, but you got to start somewhere. CT scans and MRIs are used in some advanced centres to determine the exact amount of VAT (visceral adipose tissue) in our body.

Thousands of studies have shown that *abdominal fat* is associated with lots of health problems. Why? Because the main organs of the body—including the liver, heart, main artery aorta (which supplies blood to major parts of the body)—are all in the abdominal area, and abdominal fat will compress this artery, resulting in hypertension and may also *lead to heart diseases*, indigestion, and *diabetes*.

Measure your waistline, and look at the prescribed figures below.

	Recommended waist measurement Caucasian race	South East Asia and Indian subcontinent
For men	40 inches (102 centimetres)	35.5 inches (90 centimetres)
For women	35 inches (88 centimetres)	32 inches (82 centimetres)

Anyone's waist measuring above these values have shown increased health risks, and you cannot take it casually if your waist is bloated above these figures; otherwise, you will surely end up a casualty.

Another test we commonly do is BMI (body mass index).

Oh, come on, you already know what it is and about its classification. I think everyone who is eyeballing this book knows what it is. It's just a passing reference of what you already know.

The formula is simple.

$$BMI = \text{weight in kilograms}/(\text{height in metres})^2$$

Table 1 The international classification of adult underweight, overweight, and obesity according to BMI

Classification	BMI (kg/m^2)	
	Principal cut-off points	Additional cut-off points
underweight	<18.50	<18.50
severe thinness	<16.00	<16.00
moderate thinness	16.00–16.99	16.00–16.99
mild thinness	17.00–18.49	17.00–18.49
normal range	18.50–24.99	18.50–22.99
		23.00–24.99
overweight	≥25.00	≥25.00
pre-obese	25.00–29.99	25.00–27.49
		27.50–29.99
obese	≥30.00	≥30.00
obese class I	30.00–34.99	30.00–32.49
		32.50–34.99
obese class II	35.00–39.99	35.00–37.49
		37.50–39.99
obese class III	≥40.00	≥40.00

Source: Adapted from WHO 1995, WHO 2000, and WHO 2004.

We at our clinic in North India take BMI values greater than 23 as *overweight* because it was quoted in so many researches that the international value of 25 doesn't hold true for Indian and other south Asian population because of lesser muscle weight in south Asia compared to rest of the world. And now, even the government of India has recalibrated the values of BMI, and according to new recommendations, BMI greater than 23 should be considered as overweight. It was implemented in 2011.

The first article that I read about it was back in 2001. 'BMI does not accurately predict overweight in Asian Indians in northern India' (quoted in *British Journal of Nutrition*, 86 (2001), 105–112, Department of Medicine and Department of Biostatistics, All India Institute of Medical Sciences, New Delhi 110029, India).

How Can I Measure My Body Fat?

The best way to measure your body fat is by getting your *body composition* done.

Before we discuss the methods used for measuring fat, let's find out what our body is made of. What is the composition of our body?

Interesting studies were done where males (both *lean* and *obese*) were used to estimate body composition differences. Scientists found that the *water percentage* in *lean people* was *more* than their fat percentage compared to heavier individuals.

The graph below shows two males of the same height 5 feet 9 inches and having body weights 70 kilograms and

100 kilograms respectively. The BMI of these males were 22 and 32 as calculated.

I want you to notice the difference in the macronutrient and water content in them.

Clearly the difference is in the fat and water content.

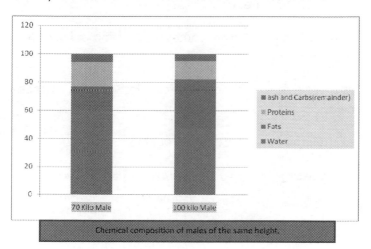

Chemical composition of males of the same height.

Methods of Detecting Fat Percentage

There are a few methods to access fat percentage, and they are:

- hydrostatic weighing (the oldest method of fat detection)
- skin fold measurements (only experts can do it as human errors are very high and results can vary greatly)

- bioelectric impedance machines (the most common assessment method; you can get it in a health store near you)
- DXA (dual-energy X-ray absorptiometry) method.
- magnetic resonance imaging and computerized tomography (which can clearly indicate thickness and volume of fat tissue).

So the next question that comes to our mind is, *how much fat is too much?*

Fat percentage in an individual can determine the fitness levels.

Let's see this in tabulated form below.

According to American Council on Exercise (for age 18 to 50)

Classification	Men (Body Fat %)	Women (Body Fat %)
essential	3–5	10–13
athletes	6–13	14–20
fit but not athletic	14–17	21–24
acceptable	18–23	25–29
obese	>24	>30

What about the Number of Fat Cells or the Size of Fat Cells in an Overweight Person? Do We Humans Have the Same Number of Fat Cells?

Increased *fats* in the body happens in two ways.

1. Hypertrophy is the filling of fat in existing fat cells.
2. Hyperplasia is the increase in number of *fat* cells in our body.

1. Hypertrophy and inflammation: There is an upper limit to the quantity of fat the fat cells can hold. Just like overinflated balloons, overfilled fat cells can burst, causing micro injuries and thus initiating inflammatory response in your body. These circulating inflammatory chemicals throughout the body are a part of the *reason* you sometimes don't lose weight *even after avoiding high-calorie food* and despite keeping energy balance by exercises and diet.
2. Hyperplasia: It is found that as you accumulate more fat, *more fat cells* are formed in your body, making weight loss even more difficult.

Scientists did some interesting studies on the amount of fat cells in varied groups of people. They did biopsy sampling of various regions of the body and counted the number of fat cells. Their research showed a strong association of being lean and having fewer numbers of fat cells as opposed to *fatty* people who had up to *ten* times more fat cells.

Interesting numbers that came out in these scientific studies were:

- An average *person* has around 27 to 30 billion fat cells in the body.
- For a mildly to moderately obese person, the number of cells can go up to 60 billion fat cells (i.e. double the number of fat cells)!

- • Now digest this. In an extremely obese person, the number can go up to 300 billion fat cells, ten times a normal person's!

That's the reason why a lot of obese cured of obesity are still at risk of gaining weight because of the greater number of fat cells that they have.

Here's another important fact: a significant number of *fat cells increase* mainly in the two phases of our life.

1. The first year of life is the time when the number of fat cells increases (my friends, your chance of being good parents and keeping your children lean and beautiful is *in the first year of your baby's life*).
2. During adolescence, again there is hyperplasia (here, the parents' job becomes difficult because of *peer pressure*).

This is the only reason we at NidSun suggest to our clients that liposuction is not so effective. It is because your body has a tendency to increase the number of fat cells again even after some of them have been sucked out through suction. Moreover, the visceral fat cannot be removed by the procedure of liposuction as it's life-threatening, and no surgeon will recommend you for visceral-fat removal through liposuction. You already know that omental or visceral fat is the main risk factor for all the diseases.

Doctors did long-term controlled studies in a man who lost a significant amount of weight, and they found something interesting.

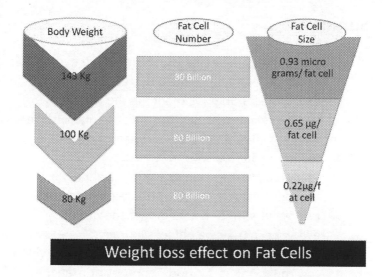

Weight loss effect on Fat Cells

As you can see in this figure, the idea of getting overweight again after some time sounds true because in people who have lost weight, the number of fat cells still remains the same as when they were obese. So if I (or any other doctor) say that you need to be extra careful with food for a few months so that weight won't come back, this makes sense.

All's Good, But What Is the Reason for the Accumulation of All that Fat?

There are lots and lots of reasons—starting from eating more calorie-dense food to the lack of physical activity, pathology in your body, and genetic defects in the body; some reasons are not even known. I will discuss this topic to the *next chapter*.

Summary

- Overweight, in simple words, is having excessive quantity of fat along with a battery of disorders.
- VAT (visceral adipose tissue) is the root cause of most medical reasons, the most dangerous fat. To test VAT, you just need a measuring tape and measure your tummy girth.
- Compared to the normal height–weight table, BMI is a much more accurate measurement for health risk management and is in fact the basic tool for everyone in their weight loss journeys.
- The best way to know whether you are carrying too much fat is by body composition analysis, which is done by various methods and gives you the true picture of fatness in the body. I will recommend everyone to get their anthropometry measurements done by a doctor or weight management centre near you. But I am assuming that if you are reading this book, you have already exhausted the self-help mode.
- Fat cells number and size is another dimension you need to know as cell number is inevitably higher in obese people, 10 times more fat cells. So comparing obese with lean people in terms of food intake is foolish! A fatty person has more fat cells, and they are much more efficient in storing fat compared to lean people. Again this is more complex than how I've explained it, but I am oversimplifying here so that you can understand it.

Chapter 3

What Causes Fat Pile-Up in Us?

I believe that it is the 'survival of the fittest' that works everywhere, and God has given this unique power to every human, including you and me, for us to use this thinking cap or the cortex, which makes us aware of things, analyse situations, and conceptualize the things that have been discovered for a better future and for better outcomes. Our lifetime won't be enough to know fully the mysteries of the human body, but then that's the pursuit of good health for all of us. The scientist and doctors should work and are working in harmony to completely solve this maze of fat.

So I am starting this journey with what is a well-known fact.

We all know that the amount of body fat in a person is directly related to the chances of developing chronic diseases, like diabetes, HTN, heart problems, hormone imbalance, etc.

Reaching a healthy weight and *staying* at it is a long-term challenge and certainly a difficult goal for everyone—me, you, everyone. The good thing, however, is that reducing weight to a healthy range will lower your risk of serious health problems by as much as 95 per cent. With the right treatment and motivation, it's possible to lose weight and lower your risk of long-term diseases, which I think is worth your efforts and consideration.

But are we not talking about superficial things only? I mean, _what is the reason for weight gain in the first place?_

Let's explore this inquisitive question that comes out of that gray matter of ours.

Your weight is the result of many *factors*. These include:

- environment
- family history and genetics
- metabolism (energy catabolism and anabolism)
- behaviour or habits
- culture
- psychology
- technology
- yoyo dieting
- lack of trust
- physical activity
- processed food and much more.

There are some *factors you can't change* (at least, not with the present scientific knowledge), such as:

- family history
- your genes
- biochemical deficits in your body.

But you have the *power to change* other factors, such as your *food* and *lifestyle* given the fact that you are physiologically in sound condition (in other words, free from chronic disease) and you are in harmony with your body and environment!

There are many exceptions to this rule of good food and good lifestyle. For example, if you have a good diet and are exercising and still not losing weight, then you definitely need professional help from a weight loss clinic or your GP as the problem may be more than skin-deep!

As the title of my book suggests, I am sure that you already know quite a few steps to prevent or treat obesity. Healthy eating, keeping calorie counts, doing physical activities **to limit** the amount of time that you're inactive are the things that, I suppose, you know. Basically, you are already aware of how to keep that energy balance for weight loss; that is the very first reason to weight gain, right? Wrong. Absolutely wrong. You wouldn't have picked up this book if you were successful with these strategies because there is much more than that!!

Weight-loss therapies, medicines, and surgery are some options for people who need to lose weight if lifestyle changes aren't enough. That's what most of knowledgeable people know. And sometimes even these don't succeed.

The question that pops out of our gray matter is 'What can I do beyond that?'

Now as I was writing this chapter, I thought of sharing a real story with you, and trust me, you won't forget it. Yes, it certainly is worth your precious time. Five years ago, an elderly female came to me for losing weight. At that time, most of my patients were referred by my father, who is a well-known cardiologist in our region (it takes a long time for people to have confidence in a doctor). So this elderly female, Miss Devi, was then seventy-one years old, a diabetic type 2 and was getting insulin injections two times in a day. She was 5 feet 4 inches tall and weighed 108 kilograms that time, and she couldn't walk. She also had frequent mild angina attacks, for which she was under medication given by my father.

When she first came to me, I was like 'Oh my god, what should I do with her? Where do I start? How will I be able to help her?' I was really scared to help her lose weight because of her multiple medical problems. I couldn't prescribe her any medication. Her triglycerides were skyrocketing. She had severe osteoarthritis on both knees. She was on a stretcher, so any kind of physical activity was almost impossible. She had angina, she had diabetes, she had asthma. Her liver functions were bad. She had varicose veins. Her urea and albumin had crossed the upper mark.

The bottom line was that only two things were fine in her reports—her thyroid functions and her will power to lose weight and deepest desire to walk again. And it was her desire to walk again that gave me hope that if she was not giving up on me, why should I give up on her? So I did what I could for her to the best of my knowledge. The first step for me was that I got her anthropometric measurements done, and I put her on a VLCD (very-low-calorie diet) and some vitamin pills along with ultrasound therapies, physiotherapy exercises by our therapists, and some psychotherapy sessions.

The initial six days, as far as I remember, were very tough on her, and she used to call me up almost every four to five hours for suggestions and queries. Then she settled down, and she began to tolerate the very-low-calorie diet. With VLCD, there is always a risk, and you should make sure that you have good reasons to lose weight because a low-calorie diet has harmful effects, but I had to do something rather than let my patient die a slow but a surely painful crippled death. So with the help of her family and the supervision of our doctors' team, we kept on going.

In her case, renal failure and ketoacidosis were my main concern, so I was monitoring those conditions continuously along with ECGs every second day for the first week. And she used to come regularly for her weight loss treatments, once in ten days, and this kept on going for four months.

You guessed it right. She came out as a winner. Soon she was on crutches from a wheelchair, and believe me, it meant a lot to her. 'I never imagined that I could be mobile so fast,' she said, and tears rolled down her cheeks. Even I had wet eyes when she said that.

Walking, instead of her family members pushing her on a wheelchair, to my office was itself motivating enough for her to carry on. After forty days, I withdrew VLCD and started giving her a 1,200-to-1,400-calorie diet with some varied food choices along with therapies, and believe me, she was off 50 per cent of her prescription medicine within those four months and finally reached 71 kilograms from 108 kilograms.

On her last weight loss session at my clinic, she cried and said, 'I am now in a dream world where I can walk and do normal household things just like I used to do twenty years back. I have a second life.' Now if you go to her home, she is running and is very active, and the only medication she is taking is an antihypertensive drug along with oral antidiabetic medication and nothing else. It was a real boost to me as well because I had just started my weight loss practice that time. I get goosebumps when I think about that transformation. That was the day when I realized the importance of my work as a preventive doctor. That incidence gave me first-hand experience of how weight loss can change someone's life for good, and that's the driving force for me to help more people. It was beginner's luck for a weight loss doctor, you might say!

The picture was not a happy ending, however, and soon after this dream, there were many failures in my career where I couldn't help my patients in weight loss despite all dietary changes and lifestyle modifications—obviously, the first line of obesity treatment we all give. But this energy balance equation works only on 40 to 45 per cent of patients. The question that haunts me is 'What about the rest, the 55 per cent of them?'

In the last five years of my weight loss practice, I have discovered that being overweight and managing weight is a much more **puzzling crossword** than any other chronic disease management. Before I discuss the rocket science of weight loss, let's quickly go through the well-known **causes of o**verweight and *obesity*.

1. Energy Balance

A positive energy balance most often causes overweight and obesity. Energy balance means energy that you give your body in the form of food (energy *in*) and energy consumed by your body in the form of metabolism and physical work (energy *out*).

Energy *in* is the amount of energy you get from food and drinks. Energy *out* is the amount of energy your body uses for things like breathing, digesting, heart function, brain function, kidney function, your activity of moving around, etc. Technically, the basal metabolic rate (BMR) of your body is energy out if you have a sedentary life.

To maintain a healthy weight, *ideally* your energy *in* and energy *out* have to balance every day. But *practically*, it's the balance over time that helps you maintain weight.

Let's assume that you have the same amount of food intake as your metabolic rate; theoretically, if you achieve it, over time your weight stays the same, and you live happily ever after!

Food (energy)

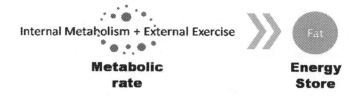

Overweight and obesity happens over time when your calorie intake is more than your metabolic rate, or it can be framed as your metabolic rate is lower compared to the food that you consume every day.

2. Lifestyle

Experts who believe in this cause of obesity say that the New Age is one of the main reasons for all of us spending hours in front of TVs and computers, doing work, schoolwork, and leisure activities. In fact, more than two hours a day of regular TV viewing or Net-surfing time has been linked to overweight and obesity all over the world.

Other genuine reasons (and excuses) for not being active include:

- using your *car* instead of walking even if you can walk

- no physical demands at work or at home because of *modern technology* and conveniences
- lack of *physical education* classes in schools for children.

People who are inactive are more likely to gain weight because they don't burn up the calories that they take in the form of food (both solid and liquid foods).

If I put it in the energy balance equation, it makes sense.

food – metabolic rate (reduced physical activity has obviously metabolic ⬇ rate) = increased fat

3. Genes and Family History

Genes have a big role in making you bloat, but genes don't make you fat literally. They contribute to your weight gain process in a way, something like this: You might have noticed a difference in the weight of individuals given the same calorie diet, especially siblings, family members, you and your friends, and everyone around you.

A genetically susceptible individual will gain more weight compared to others. Overweight/obesity tends to run in families. Your chances of being overweight are greater if one or both of your parents are overweight or obese. Even that is a complex factor being oversimplified and cannot be accused as the only factor for weight gain Why? Because I have seen a number of overweight females reducing weight after marriage through a change of external environment, and they always complained that it was their genes.

Our genes may affect the amount of fat we store in our body. Our genes even decide where on the body we carry the extra fat. The thing that should be kept in mind is that families also share food, physical activities, and habits, so this strong link between genes and environmental factors should be ruled out before we blame our genes.

My argument in favour of this is by giving example of children who adopt the habits of their parents. A child who has overweight parents who tend to eat high-calorie food and are physically less active will likely become overweight too. Why? Because for them, their parents are their role models—at least, before they reach their teenage years, where the story is different.

However, if the whole family adopts healthy food and physical activity becomes a part of their daily routine, the chance of their children being overweight or obese is reduced. If you remember, I mentioned in the previous chapter that in the first year of life and then in their adolescent years, the number of fat cells increase if you are overfed compared to children who have a balanced diet.

This argument of mine somewhat answers the question of why there are some families where almost every member is obese. As I told you, obesity is a difficult puzzle.

4. Role of Leptin in Weight Gain

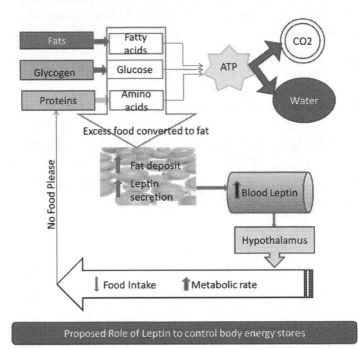

Proposed Role of Leptin to control body energy stores

Leptin is another buzzword in the medical field these days. I have tried to make a flow chart to explain the basic theory of leptin. According to this theory of leptin, it controls our food intake and metabolic rate as well. Scientists were able to find a few cases in the obese population who were deficient in leptin, and when they were given leptin, they showed good results and lost weight.

So it seems that leptin has a promising future for being studied as a factor for obesity. Before you start looking for leptin deficiency in your body, let me tell you that most of the studies done on this topic have shown that a lot of obese, on the other hand, have a very high blood concentration of leptin, which makes leptin as one of the causes for obesity but not the only one.

5. Health Conditions

As you all know, there are some hormone problems that are directly responsible for causing overweight and obesity, such as hypothyroidism, Cushing's syndrome, and polycystic ovarian syndrome (PCOS). As I am a doctor who loves to explain to my patients the root cause of their overweight problems, I cannot not tell you about these problems before we move on.

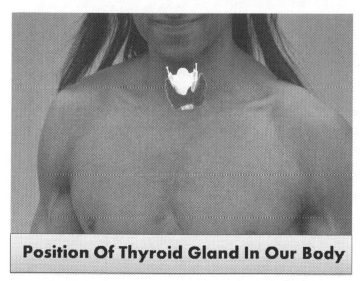

Position Of Thyroid Gland In Our Body

Hypothyroidism is a condition in which the thyroid gland doesn't make enough thyroid hormone. Lack of the thyroid hormone *thyroxine* will slow down your metabolism and cause weight gain. You'll also feel tired and weak if you have deficiency of this hormone. Doctors will tell you that you have reduced blood pressure and you might feel more heat or cold compared to a normal person because even thermoregulation in your body is hampered.

Cushing's syndrome is a condition in which the body's adrenal glands make too much of the hormone *cortisol*. Cushing's syndrome also can develop if a person takes high doses of certain medicines, such as prednisone, for long periods.

People who have Cushing's syndrome gain weight, have upper-body obesity, a rounded face, fat around the neck, and thin arms and legs.

PCOS is a condition that affects about 5–10 per cent of women of childbearing age. My every third patient suffers from PCOS. Women who have PCOS often are obese; they have excess hair growth and have reproductive problems and other health issues due to high levels of hormones called androgens (equivalent of testosterone).

I have taken up these diseases in detail in later chapters.

6. Medicines

Certain medicines may cause you to gain weight. These medicines include some *corticosteroids*, antidepressants, and *seizure* medicines.

These medicines can slow the rate at which your body burns calories, increases your appetite, and also makes your body retain water. All these factors can lead to weight gain.

7. Environmental Factors

Our environment encourages obesity in the following ways:

- *Food advertising*. Our world is full of advertisements from food divisions of MNCs. Often, children are the targets of advertising high-calorie, high-fat snacks and sugary drinks. The goal of these ads is to sway people to buy these high-calorie foods, and often they do. And then there are countless fat-free, sugar-free foods. They might be good in some cases, but it is our tendency to want more of them because they have low satiety (how much a food satisfies your hunger).

- *Work schedules*. People often say that they don't have time to be physically active because of long work hours and time spent commuting, and that's true in many cases.
- *Oversized food portions*. We are surrounded by huge food portions in restaurants, fast-food places, filling stations, movie theatres, supermarkets, and even at home. Some of these meals for *one* can feed two or more people. Eating large portions means too much energy *in*. Over time, this will cause weight gain if it isn't balanced with physical activity. Don't forget that 'buy one, get one free' makes us greedy, so much so that we don't even care whether we are hungry or not.

- *Lack of safe places for recreation*. Not having park areas, trails, sidewalks, and *affordable* gyms makes it hard for people to be physically active in so many metros.
- *Peer pressure*. This has a great effect on our weight not only in children but in adults too! My patients frequently say, 'I have to take liquor just to be socially active.' And statistics have shown time and again that more than *15 per cent* of social drinkers become habitual drinkers, and that itself is a burden to everyone in the society.
- *Lack of healthy foods*. Some people don't live in neighbourhoods that have supermarkets selling healthy foods, such as fresh fruits and vegetables. And for some people, these healthy foods are too costly. Even in India, *food inflation* is increasing only for fresh fruits, fresh vegetables, and pulses, not the packed stuff; in fact, processed food is cheaper to buy than fresh food. I sometimes fail to do the math behind it. Just think about it. Processed food is made of what they claim to be natural food, and we all know that in processing food, a lot of it is wasted, so how on earth is raw food costlier than the processed one! Do these big companies do the pricing somewhere else?

8. Emotional Factors

It is a big topic, and I have dedicated the whole chapter 8 to cover the length and breadth of this factor. *Emotional overeating* will lead to weight gain and may cause overweight/obesity, cascading the problem to new depths. Some people gain weight when they *stop smoking*. One reason is that food often tastes and smells better after quitting smoking. Another reason is because nicotine raises the rate at which your body burns calories, so you burn fewer calories when you stop smoking. However, smoking is a serious health risk, and quitting is more important than possible weight gain. To me, smoking and even *alcoholism* is just a part of emotional eating which I have discussed with emotions in some later chapter.

9. Menopause and Ageing

Menopause plays an important role in weight gain. Many women gain around 6 to 10 kilograms during menopause and accumulate more *fat around the waist* than they did before. Body structure changes occur because of lack of the hormone oestrogen. So fat starts accumulating around the waist. As you get older, you tend to lose muscle, especially if you're physically less active. Muscle loss can slow down the rate at which your body burns calories. If you don't reduce your calorie intake or increase your physical activity as you get older, you may gain weight.

Recently in India, AIIMS (All India Institute of Medical Sciences) reported that more than 50 per cent of urban females were hypertensive, which means *every second female* is hypertensive in metropolitan cities like Delhi!

There was another study which revealed that *67 per cent* of affluent women in urban India were overweight. The data is very similar to US or Britain, and it is disturbing for the nation as a whole. All these studies included females of childbearing age. It's all thanks to obesity that we don't even have to wait till menopause to get obese and have obesity-related complications.

10. Pregnancy

During pregnancy, women tend to gain weight so that their babies get proper nourishment and develop normally. Women tend to have a lot more calories than required; at least, that's what I have seen in my patients here in North India. After giving birth, some women find it real hard to lose weight. This may lead to overweight or obesity. In my clinical practice till date, *7 per cent of my patients* fall in this post-pregnancy overweight category.

11. Lack of Sleep

Yes, it is a fact that lack of sleep can cause increased fat. Studies show that people who sleep less are more likely to be overweight or obese. For example, people who reported sleeping five hours or less a night were much more likely to become obese compared to people who slept seven to eight hours.

> Sleep well and shed weight!
>
> People who sleep either more (like I do, which is a lot) or lesser than seven hours a day (afternoon naps are included, mind you) have an increased risk for cardiovascular disease, according to a new study done in some medical universities in the US.
>
> Sleeping fewer than five hours a day more than doubles your risk of being diagnosed with angina, coronary heart disease, or heart attack or stroke.

In my case, I sleep ten hours with my afternoon naps, so I am safe, right? Yes? No.

Sleeping more than eight hours also increases your risk of cardiovascular diseases; more than nine hours of sleep results in a 50 per cent increase in the risk of metabolic disease. Oh no, even I am not safe. Damn.

The daily news reports:

> The most at-risk group were adults under 60 years of age who slept five hours or less a night. They increased their risk of developing cardiovascular disease more than threefold . . . Women who skimped on sleep . . . were more than two-and-a-half times as likely to develop cardiovascular disease. all you working women who actually sleep less should note this . . . get some sound sleep.

When you are sleep-deprived, your body decreases production of leptin, the hormone that tells your brain there is no need for more food. At the same time, it also increases levels of ghrelin, a hormone that triggers hunger, which is the reason for your night cravings.

So now you know why you start having hunger pangs in the evening, the time you should in fact be having less food and more control over hunger. Mysteries of the body, I guess! (From our blog archive)

There are more causes than I have mentioned here and have discussed in future chapters as well. In fact, there are hundreds of causative factors for obesity and many theories postulated on them.

What Are the Health Risks of Being Fat?

Having fat on your body is not a sin by morality standards, but it has some bad effects and known bad effects, which you already know, but I have to discuss them to make you understand better the rocket science of fat.

'What health risks are you talking about? Isn't it's just about looking good?' said one of my patients. Of my patients who come for weight loss at our clinic, 40 to 45 per cent do it only for *aesthetic reasons*. I know it's a boring topic for those who haven't yet experienced ill health caused by obesity, but I am not here to tell you all good stories. I need to be strong enough to bare the raw facts that I believe to be true, although I am trying to make them as interesting as possible, so that you'll understand them and thus plan your future in a better way in light of knowledge rather than the darkness of ignorance.

Being overweight/obese isn't a cosmetic problem for so many of us because half of us might already be suffering from some of the repercussions of being overweight. Excess fat in our body increases the *risk for many diseases* and conditions.

Cardiovascular Diseases

Coronary heart disease (CHD) is a condition in which plaque builds up inside the coronary arteries. These arteries supply oxygen-rich blood to your heart. This plaque is made up of fat, cholesterol, calcium, antibodies, and clots.

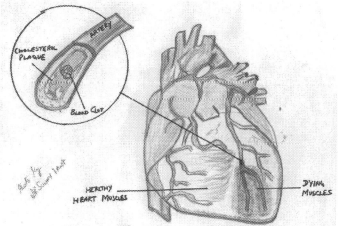

**Diagram Showing Fat deposition
In Heart (coronary) Artery resulting in Heart Attack**

Plaque can narrow or block the coronary arteries and reduce blood flow to the heart muscle. This can cause chest pain or discomfort, which we term as angina or a heart attack. Obesity is one of the main reasons leading to heart failure. This is a serious condition in which your heart can't pump enough blood to meet your body's needs.

Type 2 Diabetes

Diabetes is a disease in which the body's blood sugar level is too high. Normally, the body breaks down food into glucose and then carries it to cells throughout the body.

The cells use the hormone insulin as a key for the doors on the surface of cells so that glucose is allowed to enter through them and eventually provide energy. But there is an exception, brain! The brain is the master of the body and doesn't need insulin as a transporter of glucose like other parts of the body.

In type 2 diabetes, the body's cells *don't use insulin properly*. At first, the body reacts by making more insulin, a condition called hyperinsulinaemia. Over time, however, the body can't make enough insulin to control its blood sugar level because of *exhausted β cells* of the pancreas, and blood sugar levels rise, rapidly causing diabetes.

Diabetes is a leading cause of early death along with CHD, stroke, kidney disease, and blindness. Most people who have type 2 diabetes are *overweight*, or I should say that most overweight people have a much higher risk of getting diabetes even if they have no family history of diabetes.

Hypertension

Blood pressure is the force with which *blood pushes against the walls* of the arteries as the heart pumps out blood. If this pressure rises and stays high over time, it can damage your body in many ways. Your chances of having high blood pressure are greater if you're overweight/obese, especially people with more *abdominal fat*.

Stroke

Just like heart attack, being overweight or obese can *lead to build-up of plaque in arteries* not only in the heart but in the *brain* too. Eventually, an area of plaque can rupture, causing a blood clot to form at the site. If the clot is close to your brain, it can block the flow of blood and oxygen to your brain and cause a stroke. The risk of having a stroke rises with the rise of fat in your body.

Dyslipidemia

If you're overweight or obese, you have an increased risk of having abnormal levels of blood fats. These include high levels of triglycerides and LDL cholesterol (known as bad fats) and low levels of HDL (good fats) cholesterol.

Abnormal levels of these blood fats are an important risk factor for CHD.

Some Types of Cancer

Being overweight or obese **raises** the risk of colon, breast, endometrial, and gall bladder cancers.

Degenerative Joint Diseases

Osteoarthritis is a common joint problem of the knees, hips, and lower back. The condition occurs if the tissue that protects the joints wears away. People with extra weight can put more pressure and wear down their joints much faster, causing a lot of pain and discomfort.

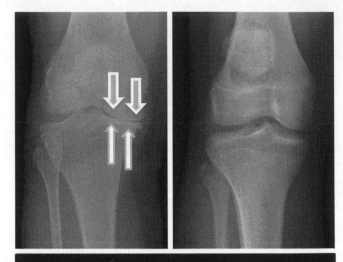

Arrows Showing Degeneration of Knee in Left Compared to normal Knee on Right side Where there is sufficient gap between the joints

Sleep Apnoea

Sleep apnoea is a common disorder in which you have one or more pauses in breathing or shallow breaths while you sleep. The reason for sleep apnoea in a person is fat stored around the neck. This can narrow the airway, making it hard to breathe.

Reproductive Problems

Obesity can cause menstrual irregularity and infertility in women (PCOS).

> Losing weight may help eliminate PCOS.

> The most important thing an individual can do if they have polycystic ovary syndrome

is to try to lose weight, which happens to be a very challenging job. Weight loss helps relieve symptoms by reducing the high levels of insulin in the body. Reducing insulin levels will lead to a reduction in testosterone, and this will help to reduce the symptoms of the condition. Weight loss can be difficult for people with polycystic ovary syndrome. It is best achieved by healthy eating and regular exercise. If you are finding it difficult to lose weight despite of exercises and a good diet, it would be wise to seek advice from us at NidSun or go to your GP.

Even if you lose weight, it is important to maintain a healthy lifestyle with regular exercise and to give up smoking if you currently smoke.

If you have been told you have PCOS (in fact, most of my patients already know they have this problem), you may feel frustrated or sad. You may also feel relieved that at last there is a reason and treatment for the problems you have been having, especially if you have had a hard time keeping a normal weight or you have excess body hair, acne, or irregular periods. Having a diagnosis without an easy cure can be difficult. However, it is important for girls with PCOS to know they are not alone. Your doctor, who knows a lot about PCOS and is someone you feel comfortable talking to, is very important. Keeping a positive attitude and working on a healthy lifestyle even when results seem to take a long time is very important too! Many girls with PCOS tell us that talking with a counsellor at NidSun about their concerns can be very helpful.

Also, it is important to follow up regularly with your doctor and make sure you take all the necessary lifestyle changes in your stride, lessening your chance of getting diabetes or other health problems. Because you have a slightly higher chance of developing diabetes, your fitness experts at NidSun may suggest that you have your blood sugar tested once a year or have a glucose challenge test every few years. Quitting smoking (or never starting) will also improve your overall health. Together we can fight this problem. ☺ (Nidhi Mohan Kamal, from our blog archive)

Gallstones

Gallstones are hard pieces of stone-like material that form in the gall bladder. They're mostly *made of cholesterol*. Gallstones can cause referred pain in upper abdomen, shoulder, or back pain.

People who are overweight or obese have an increased risk of having gallstones. Also, being overweight may result in an enlarged gall bladder that doesn't work right.

Children and Teens

Overweight and obesity also increase the health risks for children and teens. Type 2 diabetes was once rare in children, but increasing numbers of children are developing the disease. We have had thirty-two cases of obese teens with type 2 diabetes who had come for weight loss treatments.

Also, **overweight children** have very high tendencies to become overweight or **obese as adults** with high disease risks.

So you know that being overweight is not only aesthetically bad but bad for your health as well. My friend, awareness is the key to good health. I will start my rocket science of weight loss in the next few chapters, so stay connected.

Summary

1. **The causes of being fat** are numerous, most of them being positive energy balance, genetic factors, hormonal imbalance, age, menopause, environmental factors, emotional factors, pregnancy, lack of sleep, post-addiction time, alcohol, medication, and a lot more.
2. **Leptin deficiency** was also considered as an important cause of obesity, but scientists have found overproduction of leptin in a lot of overweight people, so even that theory doesn't work on every one.

3. Obesity represents a **medical condition** that is a cocktail of various conditions such as dyslipidemia, cardiac abnormalities, hypertension, stroke, type 2 diabetes, hypothyroidism, insulin resistance, glucose intolerance, joint problems, digestion problems, and even cancer. They are directly related to being overweight, and awareness to all these is the key to prevention.

4. Prevention is the most underrated remedy to most of the chronic diseases.

Chapter 4

Introduction to Categorization of Overweight

Through my journey as a weight loss expert, I have eyeballed hundreds of books on weight loss, obesity, diet and nutrition, health and fitness, exercises recommendations, kinesiology, anthropometry, biomechanics of the human body, and so many more along with regular medical subjects that we all doctors have to study. Many doctors, fitness experts, diet experts, and patients have helped me in gaining all that knowledge, and still my success rate for helping people losing weight is only 80 per cent. What about the 20 per cent who couldn't benefit from our knowledge and expertise?

If I blame my patients for not complying to the advised diet, exercise, and therapy programs during weight loss therapies, I won't improve my procedures, and I am sure that my organization will stroll. That 20 per cent of our patients drive us to know more, study more, attend more seminars, make more teachers, and learn more, and I wish that I would never pretend to be perfect and be like any other scientist. I wish to remain a child in learning, always inquisitive and always absorbing, always hungry.

Through that journey, we came up with some discoveries, improvisations, and observations. Based on these, we formulated some information and chunked them in words and sentences for others to explore the journey to losing weight. This is just a background for you to warm you up before starting this chapter.

There are a lot of definitions and classifications of obesity, the most popular being the stages of overweight:

- mild obesity
- moderate obesity
- morbid obesity based on BMI, fat per cent, overall weight.

I wish that obesity classification were that simple.

I have broadly categorized overweight into four types of patients based on our practical experiences and customization of therapies for weight management in individuals, but there are people who overlap in more than one category.

I want you to have a better understanding about the reasons for your obesity and choosing the appropriate treatment and diet that suit your needs and are tailor-made for you.

The four categories of overweight/obese patients that we have segregated for clinical and practical *ataraxy* are as follows:

a. ignorant obese
b. diseased obese
c. food addict obese
d. knowledgemongering obese.

I will take all the four categories as separate chapters for better comprehension. So let's start with ignorant obesity in this chapter and the rest of the three in subsequent chapters and try to find your specific category.

Ignorant Obesity

Almost *60 per cent* of the obese population falls in this category—all those who have recently changed their diet or have come from rural areas into an urban environment and those who were not used to high-calorie concentrated food and those who have no medical problems being ignorant about diet, exercise, and awareness of medical complications related to obesity.

The ignorant obese form the main chunk of overweight people.

In this particular category, the main *causes of weight gain* are:

- positive energy balance
- lack of physical activity
- excess of liquor or supplements intake (although it is a subcategory of positive energy balance, we take it as a separate cause).

The more the number of calories consumed in the form of food, beverages, and supplements, especially if it exceeds daily body requirements (i.e. physical activity plus the basal metabolic rate of your body), the more you have a positive energy balance. I will explain this phenomenon in this chapter.

At our clinic, we have only 20 per cent of total patients who fall in this category because ignorant obese and overweight people get a lot of benefits by either reducing their diet or increasing their physical activates or both on advice of friends, gym trainers' and dieticians. For these people losing weight is very easy even with help of few weight loss tip and knowledge, they can change themselves and lose weight.

The *ignorant population can become obese* under these special circumstances:

- females who might be having a history of pregnancy related weight gain
- post-menopausal gain because of reduced BMR (basal metabolic rate)
- age-related weight gain
- illness needing bed rest.

Interestingly, if you are reading this book, you are unlikely to be in the ignorant obesity category because I assume that you already know what to eat and how much to exercise, and chances are that you are already doing everything you can to lose weight, right? But I would still like to elaborate on this topic a bit. Consider refreshing your memory.

Signs and symptoms of ignorant obesity can be the following:

1. very little knowledge about healthy foods and the concept of diet
2. very little knowledge about the concept of exercise
3. little or no knowledge about the consequences of being overweight

4. lack of exercise and excess of calories due to work pressure and socializing
5. chronic injuries and ill health requiring bed rest, leading to positive energy balance and causing weight gain.

What should be *the line of treatment* for ignorant obesity?

Treatment of ignorant obesity is awareness of the concept of diet and exercise and awareness about medical complications related to obesity. You can safely say that they are novice obese. All they need is a good diet plan and a good exercise plan, and they will gradually come to shape and shed that extra fat that was stored in hibernation or because of overnutrition or underactivity.

Lately, I have seen a lot of people who had lost weight on their own unknowingly misguide other people about losing weight and make fun of weight loss clinics, and I can understand their situation because they feel that weight loss is easy. They had done it on their own without much problem, so they want to pass the knowledge on to others. The ignorant obese may have found losing weight easy, but they should understand the diversity of situations for every single individual and that they are not representing the whole population. What about those who find it tough to lose weight? That was the fundamental reason for me to formulate a classification of obesity that works on the grounds of reality and is practically implementable.

People who fall in this category should, with the help of a family doctor's go-ahead, start some form of moderate exercise, like walking, and gradually increase exercise intensity to moderate intensity (exercises for up to one hour/day) and start taking healthier snacks and regular meals suggested by their doctor or dietician. This will make losing weight a much safer affair, and they won't need specialized clinics like ours.

This is the type of people who get maximum effect from diet counselling and exercise under the guidance of good dieticians and experienced trainers respectively. I still suggest for the ignorant obese to keep their doctors informed about the diet and exercise changes they do even if they are losing weight steadily, especially when they are recovering from chronic illness or injury.

You can go to the gym, weight loss centres (which should have a team of at least a doctor, dietician, and fitness experts if possible), recreational clubs, or you can do anything that keeps you active and get good results.

Precaution and Note

If you are planning weight loss on your own, *and* most people do it on their own for the first time anyway! Always make sure that you discuss your diet with your doctor or qualified dietician at least once so that they can suggest some corrections in your diet, making it good, wholesome, and rich in vitamins and nutrients. You can go walking or do any other physical activity, like cycling, jogging, swimming, golf, tennis, badminton, skipping, stair climbing, tracking, or joining a gym.

If your diet is good and you are doing more than thirty minutes of any physical activity along with having a physically active day, you can expect to lose 0.5-kilogram weight almost every week but not faster.

The Story of My First Patient, Who Was Ignorant Obese

By the time I reached my third year in medical school, I was the one from whom every doctor used to seek help for diet tips because everyone in the college knew that I had experimented with each and every type of diet. You name it, and I had it (liquid diet; VLCD; high-carb diet for carbohydrate loading; weight gain–weight loss diet; high-protein, low-fat, low-carb diet; Atkins diet; South Beach diet; Dr Bernstein's diet; leptin diet; GI diet; total-well-being diet; Stone Age diet; ADF diet; blood group diet; cabbage soup; HCG diet; egg diet; vegan diet). And I knew first-hand lots of positive effects and side effects of each of those diets by the end of medical school.

Some of the side effects landed me at our hospital many times. I even had diets from dieticians in our medical school. All in all, my pals were quite impressed by the way I used to transform my body to lean, muscular, or overweight. In more-technical terms, I used to have body types that are ectomorphic to ectomeso to mesomorphic to endomeso and back to ectomorphic in a matter of months.

I had a very handsome friend who was a year junior to me. One day, he came to me, absolutely intoxicated with liquor to the hilt, hardly able to walk, and he came and crashed on my bed and started crying. He said, 'My girlfriend ditched me because I am fat. Dr Sunny, will you help me lose weight?' My first weight loss patient in my third year of medical school? How could I say *no* to a fellow doctor? Not bad. I said, 'Sure, why not?' And that night around sixteen years back, I made my first official written diet plan for someone. LOL.

I made a killer diet for him with hardly 800 calories a day. For someone like my friend, who was 5 feet 11 inches and weighed 110 kilograms that time, it was like starving. To my surprise, he managed to stick to it, and because he had no medical problems, he was losing weight rapidly. All was great, and then he lost 16 kilograms in a month. I was really worried about him because he looked so weak and had started using electric stimulations in the physiotherapy department and used to run for thirty minutes. My worries were that if something happened to this guy, his parents were going to kill me and that in my experience, it was too rapid-paced for weight loss. I warned him of the problems and complications of sudden weight loss, but he said, 'I want to weigh 80 kilograms, and I will follow your diet till I reach that mark.' And guess what, he reached his target weight in three months flat, *but* with a prolapsed rectum, for which he had to be operated. But he survived without a hiccup and still loves me to be his weight loss mentor.

Guys, that was my first patient of weight loss, who made my future career clear to me. Why was I born on planet earth? To be a weight loss expert, what else? But first success, as they say, is beginner's luck.

Note and warning: Always consult your doctor before starting your weight loss plan or visit some weight loss clinic and have counselling with the doctor there. Weight lose should be at a good pace, not at a rapid pace; otherwise, you will land into some grave situation.

The Basic of Diets

Let's quickly brush through the basics of diets even though you have a good knowledge of food.

I am not going to bash or talk ill of any diet for weight loss because all the doctors, dieticians, naturopaths, and trainers who have ever come up with their unique ways of diet cocktails based on the type and health status of their clients and their experiences have done hard work in helping people and there can be an infinite number of diets that can be made according to the needs and requirements of the person undergoing fat reduction. That's the reason you should still consult your doctor before starting any drastic diet cocktail.

All diets work well, but if you restrict any one of the three macronutrients to negligible amounts for a longer time, you are bound to have trouble. There should be little variations between the ratios of carbohydrates, proteins, and fats, and no more. The balance in diet can come with the right ratios of calories from all three macronutrients, and the combinations that you can make are infinite. Some examples are:

Ratios	Carbohydrates (%)	Proteins (%)	Fats (%)
good diet	40–50	30–35	20–30
no-carbohydrate diet	2–5	40–50	40–45
high-protein diet	20	50–60	20
VLC diet (500–800 calories)	40	30	30
high-protein, high-fat diet	10	45	45
low-fat diet	55	35	10

Let's suppose your doctor or dietician suggested you a 45-35-30 diet plan of 1,300 calories for weight loss. What does that mean?

It means:

- Out of 1,300 calories, 45 per cent of that (585 calories) in your diet should come from carbohydrates, meaning you will have roughly 145 grams of carbohydrates in your diet (1 gram of carbohydrates gives you 4 calories).
- The *35* is for proteins, which means 35 per cent of the total calories are from proteins. It comes out to be 455 calories, and the amount of proteins in your diet should be 114 grams, choosing various food combinations (1 gram of protein releases 4 calories of energy, equal to carbohydrates).
- Similarly, the *30* is for fat, which means 30 per cent of calories in your diet will come from fats, making it 390 calories coming from fat. This means your diet has 43 grams of fat. Don't be shocked; values are less because 1 gram of fat releases 9 calories of energy.

Again, it won't be that simple a calculation, which I have shown in this table, because your dietician will take care of your health and make sure you have carbohydrates from a variety of sources, like whole grains, pulses, beans, cereals, and vegetables. Yes, a lot of people think that carbs are only in cereals and that other food groups don't have it. That's a myth.

The light of knowledge destroys ignorance, doesn't it?

Your diet experts will discourage you to have any refined white carbohydrates, like sugar, because simple carbs disturb the delicate blood sugar balance in your body.

Your diet expert will also make sure that you get healthy and essential fats from both animal and plant sources in the right combination and you don't have any hydrogenated or trans-fat-containing food products. And they will also ensure that your food portions are not in excess.

Sometimes even healthy foods in excess can increase weight like crazy.

> Healthy foods can increase your weight, so be careful

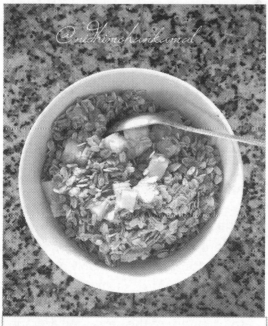

Healthy FOOD in excess can make us FAT

Yesterday, I had a patient who has gained 0.5-kilogram weight in the last one week as she has started using olive oil!

Read the full blog before you say or think anything.

- Olive oil is a hit these days, and there is a reason behind that. It is high in monounsaturated fats, which help keep your cholesterol levels in check and keeps your heart healthy. Now what you should be careful about is that 1 tablespoon of olive oil has 125 calories. Switch from your normal oil to olive oil (rather than add it as an extra to your diet as my patient was doing), and please don't exceed 2 tablespoons/day. More of healthy food is also sometimes really bad for your health. An example is my patient; she was shocked to see her weight going up 0.5 kilogram just because of this mistake. Fortunately, we were able to detect it, and she is back on track and getting ready for her wedding in the coming month.
- Another blunder that happens with some people is the quantity of the health cereal muesli! Yeah, the healthy, crunchy muesli is rich in fibres and minerals like zinc and magnesium and better than some highly processed cereals which are high in sodium and bad for your heart; however, you should be careful again about the quantity of this cereal. An average bowl of muesli with double-toned milk has 287 calories

and 4.9 grams of fat, compared to 149 calories and 1.8 grams of fat in cornflakes. And please don't have more than a 50-gram serving as this cereal is calorie-dense. Make sure that it is an unsweetened or sugar-free variety of muesli.

So next time you go for healthy meals for weight loss or maintenance, please be aware of the portions of food that go inside your body; otherwise, you will get the jolt of your life when you get on the weighing scale.

My Treatment Practice

In type A patients (ignorant obese), I usually prescribe a tried-and-tested low-fat diet, which works great with clinical modalities like ultrasound and radiofrequency for body contouring. For a good amount of weight loss, you need to have a low-fat diet, especially if you are taking these therapies. For my patients who ask only for a diet plan, I prefer giving them a balanced diet with all the macronutrients in the right ratios of 40-30-30 but restrict them to a total number of calories of 1,100–1,700/day, depending upon the basal metabolic rate and with the condition that their medical tests are normal.

We always encourage our patients to have good and wholesome food without any time restrictions or amount of serving. They can have two meals, three meals, or the more-popular six small meals in a regular interval of time. It's their wish as long as they have food from all the food groups. Also, taking care that total number of calories consumed during the day doesn't go beyond the recommended intake. If my patients don't have any gross clinical illnesses or joint pains, I always tell them to do some physical activity they like to do because weight loss therapies won't be with you forever. Therapies just help you like a good teacher, but it's you who has to pass the examination, not your teacher.

You have endless options to exercise and keep yourself active. By the end of this chapter, you will be exhausted by the options that I'll give you for your physical activities. Choose the one that you love.

Eating carbs at night makes you fat, true or false?

No roti, no rice, no pasta, no breads, no potatoes, no dal . . . no you, no me, no world. Eat carbs at night, and they will remain in your system because, at that time, you are sleeping and your metabolism is slow so it will be converted into fat. Does that mean I can hog like a pig before 6 p.m.? False, false, false.

If by any chance you are losing weight by cutting carbs at night, that's because you are cutting the total number of calories out of one of your main meals. Interestingly, that can be any meal, irrespective of it being your breakfast, lunch, dinner, morning snacks, 6 p.m. to midnight. All that matters is the type of carbs and the total calories you consume in twenty-four hours.

The myth that eating carbs at night can make you fat was just another gimmick to restrict calories and had spread like a wildfire with absolutely no scientific evidence to it. We at NidSun say that evenings are the ideal time to enjoy food, and it will be foolish to stop your evening carbs unless you are extremely obese. In that case, being a doctor, I or any doctor in the whole world will certainly prescribe you with VLCD (very-low-calorie diet) because obesity is a time bomb and you have to defuse it as fast as possible before you get destroyed!

Another reason it's not a very good idea to cut your carbs at night is that eating at night, especially if you have complex carbs, can help you sleep well, but just watch the total calories throughout the day though.

The latest study which proves that eating carbs at night don't make you fat comes from Israel. Scientists in Israel summoned seventy-eight obese members of the Israeli police force for a six-month randomized clinical trial. The first group was prescribed a low-calorie diet (20 per cent protein, 30–35 per cent fat, 45–50 per cent carbohydrates, and 1,300–1,500 kilocalories) with most of the carbohydrates being served at dinner. The second group consumed a similar diet of 1,300–1,500 kilocalories except that carbohydrate intake was spread throughout the day, rather less in dinner.

What happened after six months?

The first group, who ate most of their carbohydrates at night, lost less weight. A big no, no, no>>>, they actually lost 2 kilograms more weight than the second group, who did not eat carbs at night. (From blog archive)

Exercise

I know that you know all about exercise, but just in case you forgot, let's brush through these exciting topics of activities, exercises, and workouts.

Your body has this simple rule: use it or lose it. It's not about weight loss; it's about your health. Physical activity should be there in the form of anything you like, anything you really like to do that moves you. And do it every day for thirty minutes for maintaining good health. This summarizes pretty much everything about exercise knowledge.

Let's see what is recommended by health experts. Scientists are tired of doing studies on how much of exercise is enough, and they have come up with the conclusion that if you even do ten minutes of exercise at a time just to start the routine, it is enough for improving health.

You can negotiate on things, but this is health, not a thing.

The recommended minimum levels of activity for each age group according to health departments of the US, UK, and Canada are as follows:

- children under five years old
  - o Each day, exercise should be for 180 minutes (3 hours) once a child is able to walk!
  - o For non-walkers, physical activity should be encouraged from birth, particularly through floor-based play and water-based activities in safe environments.
- children and young people (five to eighteen years old)
  - o Every day, this should include sixty minutes and up to several hours of moderate- to vigorous-intensity physical activities.
  - o Three days a week should include vigorous-intensity activities that strengthen muscles and bones.
- adults (nineteen to sixty-four years old) and older people (sixty-five plus)
  - o Each week, 150 minutes (2.5 hours) of moderate- to vigorous-intensity physical activities (and adults should aim to do some physical activities every day).
  - o Muscle-strengthening activities should also be included twice a week.

I am a sports doctor, and I love to give lists of activities to people; technically, we call it exercise prescription. So here is a nice, long list of activities you can choose from. If you haven't done them, try every one of them, and you will find what you like to do.

Moderate or vigorous exercises you might already be doing are as follows:

1. Moderate-intensity physical activities (burn 3.5 to 7 kilocalories/minute)

   - walking at a moderate or brisk pace of 5 to 6.5 kilometres/hour on a level surface
   - cycling at speed of 9 to 15 kilometres/hour
   - calisthenics (light)
   - yoga
   - gymnastics
   - general home exercises, light or moderate effort (getting up and down between floors)
   - jumping on a trampoline
   - using a stairclimber machine at a light-to-moderate pace
   - using a rowing machine with moderate effort
   - boxing (punching bag)
   - modern dancing, disco, ballet
   - table tennis
   - tennis (doubles)
   - golf (wheeling or carrying clubs)
   - basketball (shooting baskets)
   - weight training and bodybuilding using free weights
   - roller skating or in-line skating at a leisurely pace
   - playing frisbee, juggling, curling
   - cricket (batting and bowling)
   - badminton
   - archery
   - fencing

- downhill skiing (with light effort), ice skating at a leisurely pace (10 kilometres/hour or less), snowmobiling, ice sailing
- swimming (recreational, treading water), diving (springboard or platform), aquatic aerobics, waterskiing, snorkelling, surfing (board or body)—with slow, moderate effort
- canoeing or rowing a boat at less than 2 kilometres/hour, white-water rafting, sailing (recreational or competition), paddle boating, kayaking on a lake on calm water
- washing or waxing a powerboat or the hull of a sailboat
- horseback riding (general saddling or grooming a horse)
- playing on school playground equipment, moving about, swinging, climbing, or playing hopscotch, four square, dodge ball, tee-ball, hide and seek, or tetherball
- skateboarding, roller-skating or in-line skating (leisurely pace)
- playing instruments while actively moving; playing in a marching band; playing guitar or drums in a rock band, twirling a baton in a marching band, singing while actively moving about as on stage
- gardening and yard work: raking the lawn, bagging grass or leaves, digging, hoeing, light shovelling (less than 5 kilograms per minute), weeding while standing or bending, planting trees, trimming shrubs and trees, hauling branches, stacking wood, pushing a power lawnmower

- moderate housework: scrubbing the floor or sweeping an outdoor area, cleaning out the garage, washing windows, moving light furniture
- actively playing with children (walking, running, or climbing while playing with children), walking while carrying a child weighing less than 23 kilograms
- general home construction work: roofing, painting inside or outside of the house
- handwashing and waxing a car (my favourite)
- briskly walking on a level surface while carrying a suitcase or load weighing up to 23 kilograms.

2. Vigorous-intensity physical activities (burn more than 7 kilocalories/minute)

- race-walking and aerobic walking (7.5 kilometres/ hour or faster), running and jogging, walking and climbing briskly up a hill, backpacking
- mountain climbing, rock climbing
- roller-skating or in-line skating at a fast pace
- bicycling more than 17 kilometres/hour or bicycling on steep uphill terrain, stationary bicycling using vigorous effort
- calisthenics (push-ups, pull-ups, vigorous effort) and circuit weight training
- karate, judo, tae kwon do, ju-jitsu, aikido
- jumping rope, performing jumping jacks
- using a stairclimber machine at a fast pace
- using a rowing machine with vigorous effort
- using an arm-cycling machine with vigorous effort
- boxing in the ring, sparring
- wrestling (competitive)

- professional ballroom dancing (energetically), square dancing (energetically), folk dancing (energetically)
- clogging
- tennis (singles), wheelchair tennis
- football game
- basketball game
- wheelchair basketball
- soccer
- rugby
- kickball
- hockey
- handball (general or team)
- racquetball
- squash
- downhill skiing (racing or with vigorous effort), ice-skating (fast pace or speed skating), cross-country skiing, sledding, tobogganing, playing ice hockey
- canoeing or rowing more than 6.5 kilometres/hour, kayaking in white-water rapids, swimming (steady-paced laps, synchronized swimming, treading water with fast, vigorous effort), water jogging, water polo, water basketball, scuba diving
- horseback riding (trotting, galloping, jumping, in competition, playing polo)
- playing a heavy musical instrument while actively running in a marching band
- gardening and yard work: heavy or rapid shovelling (more than 5 kilograms per minute), digging ditches, carrying heavy loads, felling trees, carrying large logs, swinging an axe, hand-splitting logs, climbing and trimming trees, or pushing a non-motorized lawnmower

- shovelling heavy snow
- heavy housework: pushing furniture (40 kilograms or more), carrying household items weighing 10 kilograms or more up a flight of stairs
- shovelling coal into a stove
- standing, walking, or walking down a flight of stairs while carrying objects weighing 20 kilograms or more
- vigorously playing with children, running longer distances, or playing strenuous games with children
- race-walking or jogging while pushing a stroller designed for sport use, carrying an adult or a child weighing 12 kilograms or more
- standing or walking while carrying an adult or a child weighing 21 kilograms or more
- concrete or masonry work
- pushing a disabled car (my nightmare)
- carrying animals weighing over 23 kilograms, handling or carrying heavy animal-related equipment or tack.

If initially you don't want to do any of the long options, I recommend that you minimize your sedentary behaviour by including these effective tips:

- reducing time spent watching TV, using the computer, or playing video games
- taking regular breaks at work
- breaking up sedentary time by activities such as swapping a long bus or car journey for walking part of the way.

These are not my guidelines alone. All these are in accordance to CDC, CMO (UK), and ACSM guidelines.

'We all have become extremely sedentary, and I believe that this is one of those reasons why you are going to see those guideline numbers come down every second year,' said a health expert regarding creation of the new guidelines. I think that we should not negotiate further!

My intentions of giving you an almost infinite list of activities is to open your eyes and make you realize that there are other exercise options aside from going to the gym. I know that you don't have time for the gym, but you can move, can do these things in your office, and can do them at home. You just need to be creative to find an activity that gels with your daily routine. This is not even for weight loss; it's the bare minimum to keep up general health!

Real-Life Example

I have a patient who is working in Delhi as a general manager in MNC. She lost 4 kilograms of weight (only fat loss), and she was doing everything great and was getting good results from our clinic except for one thing—no activity. I told her to be creative and to do something about that because I won't be giving her any more therapies. She came to me after a month. She had lost another kilo on her own and told me that she had come up with an innovative way to exercise.

Now digest this. What she did was that she kept her sneakers in the car because she noted that there was at least a forty-five-minute to one-hour traffic jam at almost the same place every single day while on her way back from the office. She said, 'I take out my sneakers and go out for some rounds at a nearby park till the traffic is cleared, and that's how I do a brisk walk for thirty-five to forty minutes and go back to my chauffeur-driven car, which has covered hardly two kilometres in that time period!' That's extremely creative innovation.

I must caution you, though, don't try this idea if you drive your car; otherwise, be responsible for what will happen to your darling when you go back. Have some imagination!

Summary

- I have broadly categorized overweight into four types: ignorant obese, diseased obese, food addict obese, and knowledgemongering obese.
- In this chapter, I have covered the ignorant obese. By definition, they are those who have high-calorie concentrated food or low physical activity or both, with no medical problems, and they do it all unknowingly.
- Treatment is the awareness of the concept of diet, exercise, and awareness about medical complications related to obesity.
- There are various diets available, and they all have various ratios of carbohydrates, fats, and proteins. In this category, the best ratio would be high carbohydrates and proteins and low-fat meals, but any ratio in low calories will do the trick!
- Ideally, thirty minutes of exercise should be done every day to maintain good health. I am not even talking about weight loss here.

Chapter 5

Diseased Obese

About *10 per cent* of my patients are under this category of obesity. As the name suggests, diseased obesity is overweight/obesity condition caused by a diseases or pathology. Examples are:

- hypothyroidism
- PCOS
- viral infections
- Cushing's syndrome
- hypothalamic damage (because of injury or tumour causing damage to satiety centre)
- micronutrient deficiencies
- genetic factors like (Laurence–Moon syndrome and Prader–Willi syndrome)
- psychiatric conditions, like bulimia nervosa
- genetic hormonal deficiencies
- genetic enzyme deficiencies
- type 1 and type 2 diabetes and all other metabolic abnormalities.

Now the list I have given above has some diseases which I call dual diseases. Doctors can find out the details depending on the patient's case history. Examples of these kinds of dual diseases—or as I call them, confusion diseases—which cause obesity *or* is caused by obesity are as follows:

- type 2 diabetes
- hypothyroidism
- PCOS
- micronutrient deficiency.

If you are confused right now, don't worry, it will be cleared by the end of this chapter.

We already know that obesity is the main causative factor for diseases like:

- glucose intolerance
- insulin resistance
- type 2 diabetes
- dyslipidemia (increased triglycerides and LDL and decreased HDL)
- hypertension
- cancer
- increased risk of heart diseases
- osteoarthritis
- lower back pain
- elevated C-reactive protein
- depression
- lack of energy
- PCOD
- hypothyroidism.

As we had discussed in chapter 2, out of these risk factors caused by obesity, type 1 and type 2 diabetes, PCOS, and hypothyroidism can be presented even before you become obese; rather, they may be the reason why a person becomes obese. Now the debate of what diseases cause obesity and what diseases obesity is causing is an old one. Remember the age-old debate of whether the chick came first or the egg came first. I know that you know the answer, and the fact is that everyone knows that it is not that simple!

A careful assessment of the patient's history, symptoms, behaviours, and mental status is the first step in making a diagnosis. The complete assessment usually requires an hour and includes a thorough review of these chronic diseases in the patient and their families to determine whether the disease caused obesity or obesity led to that disease.

Let's explore these obesity-causing diseases one by one.

Hypothyroidism

Hypothyroidism is a condition in which thyroid function becomes slow. There are a number of reasons for a person to suffer from hypothyroidism. It can be autoimmune (your immune system working against your own thyroid gland).

Or it can be acquired by some external factors:

- drug inducement
- after radioiodine treatment or thyroidectomy
- iodine deficiency
- iodine excess
- anti-thyroid drugs
- some antipsychotic drugs
- excess of goitrogenic foods
- mercury toxicity.

In bodybuilders who abuse HGH (human growth hormone), IGF-1 (insulin-like growth hormone), drugs for building muscles, I have seen many subclinical hypothyroidism being developed. Bodybuilders and bikini athletes also take T3 and T4 for shedding weight and can have adverse effects on health, leading to hypothyroidism.

Mercury toxicity can also result in hypothyroidism and hence the weight gain. Heavy metals interacting with one another exaggerate the negative effects on your body. For example, the presence of lead in the diet and the atmosphere can make the weight gain effect of mercury much stronger.

If you start gaining weight, feel tired, depressed, and start having muscle pains, then your doctor may order for a detailed blood test, including the thyroid function test. Once you are detected with hypothyroidism, your doctor will prescribe you *medications* and will also tell you to avoid or reduce some foods that may reduce thyroid functioning.

We should know that many good foods like broccoli may not be good for hypothyroid patients. These foods have substances which are known as goitrogens. These goitrogens reduce iodine uptake by the thyroid gland, thus causing problems with the way your thyroid works. These foods (cooking inactivates the goitrogens) have been identified as goitrogenic foods. They include:

- soybeans (and soybean products, such as tofu, soybean oil, soy flour, soy lecithin)
- peanuts
- millet
- strawberries

- pears
- peaches
- spinach
- sweet potatoes
- broccoli
- Brussels sprouts
- cabbage
- canola
- cauliflower
- mustard greens
- radishes
- turnips.

All these foods are good, but if you have hypothyroidism, you should limit the intake of these foods and never have them raw.

PCOS

Polycystic ovary syndrome (PCOS) is a condition that affects the ovaries.

The ovaries are found in women and consist of a pair of glands which are on either side of the uterus (womb). The ovaries produce ova (eggs), which are released into the uterus once a month during the menstrual cycle. Each ovum develops in the ovary from a small swelling called a follicle. Usually, several of these follicles develop each month, but only one will produce a fully matured ovum.

Each month, at least twelve to fourteen follicles develop on the surface of the ovary. This is more than the usual. The follicles are also known as cysts, and this is how the disease gets its name: polycystic (*poly* means 'many', *cystic* refers to 'follicles') ovary syndrome.

The cysts on the ovaries are fluid sacs.

The woman will not have periods, or they will be irregular in nature.

Ovaries produce higher levels of testosterone than normally produced.

There are a number of symptoms associated with this syndrome.

- absent or irregular periods
- weight gain
- acne (spotty skin)
- hirsutism (excessive hair growth on the face and body)
- difficulties in getting pregnant
- thinning of scalp hair.

Your doctor might want you to get some *confirmatory blood tests*. These are used to measure levels of hormones, including testosterone and luteinizing hormone. This can also help to rule out alternative hormone problems that might cause periods to stop. *USG (ultra sonography)* is done to look at the surface of the ovaries. This will show whether the ovaries are enlarged and polycystic.

Accordingly, your doctor will prescribe you some *medications and exercise*.

In PCOS patients, it is *very difficult to lose weight* just by diet and exercise. A lot of my patients do lose weight but at a painfully slow pace compared to non-PCOS obese patients.

All in all, two out of ten patients suffering from PCOS quit our weight loss programme in the middle. The reason is that they only lose inches from their problem area but the weight loss is less. And now for the last one year, we have started focusing on the aggressive use of ultrasound modalities and comprehensive diets and physical activity schedules for our PCOS patients. Even then I admit that some cases of PCOS are really difficult to manage. At our weight loss clinic, we have 80 per cent success rate with PCOS cases. Patience is the key to losing weight in these cases.

Viral Infections

Researchers have identified *adenovirus 36 or Ad-36* (one adenovirus of a family of about fifty viruses that cause colds, upper respiratory infections, gastrointestinal problems, and eye inflammations and infections) in the *development of obesity* in humans and other animals.

Adenovirus 36 (Ad-36) was first described in 1980 at about the time that the prevalence of obesity began to increase. Scientists observed that obese humans had a higher prevalence of serum neutralizing antibodies to

Ad-36 (*30 per cent*) compared to lean humans (*11 per cent*), and they showed that antibody-positive obese or non-obese patients were on an average heavier compared with their antibody-negative counterparts. Similarly, scientists also observed that when human twins are detected for antibodies to Ad-36, the *antibody-positive twin had a higher body mass index due to more fat content in the body*.

Why Does Ad-36 Cause Obesity?

The speculated reason that Ad-36 causes obesity is that it *accelerates the transformation of pre-adipocytes to adipocytes* (the *hyperplasia* of fat cells, as we discussed in previous chapters) in human pre-adipocytes, so this *increase in number of fat cells* makes a person more susceptible to obesity.

Another Virus in the Scanner

In 1992, Nihil V. Dhurandhar, PhD, at the then University of Bombay, India, reported on the avian adenovirus *SMAM-1*, which caused *excessive intra-abdominal fat deposition* and paradoxically low serum cholesterol and triglyceride levels in chickens. Antibodies against SMAM-1 virus were found in ten of fifty-two humans with obesity screened in Mumbai. Those *people with antibodies* had a *significantly higher body weight* and body mass index (BMI).

In brief, researchers have found that around *30 per cent* of the people with obesity had the antibodies compared with *11 per cent* who had antibodies but had normal weight. Still a lot of research is going on for blaming viruses as one of the causes of obesity in mankind. If their studies prove to be right, the next step would be mass vaccination programs, just like we did for polio and smallpox.

Cushing's Syndrome

Cortisol is the body's main stress hormone. Cortisol is secreted by the adrenal glands in response to the secretion of adrenocorticotropic hormone (ACTH) by the pituitary. Cushing's syndrome is caused by an over secretion of ACTH by the pituitary leading to an *excess of cortisol*.

The causes of Cushing's syndrome:

1. Cushing's syndrome can result from taking an excessive amount of medication used to treat asthma, lupus, and rheumatoid arthritis among other diseases.
2. A more serious cause can be a pituitary tumour or other growth around it or maybe directly from a tumour on the adrenal glands situated above the kidneys.

People with Cushing's syndrome show symptoms like:

*   upper body obesity
*   rounded face
*   increased fat around the neck
*   thinning of arms and legs.

Children tend to be obese with slowed growth rates, purplish pink stretch marks, severe fatigue, weak muscles, high blood pressure, depression, and high blood sugar.

If your doctor suspects Cushing's syndrome, after the routine history, physical exam, and basic blood tests, she or he might ask you for more blood, saliva, and urine tests to measure the amount of serum cortisol. If those levels are high, the doctor may order a test called *dexamethasone suppression test* along with CT or MRI to determine the *presence and location of a tumour*, if suspected. It is very important to get your complete tests done as suggested by your doctor so that proper treatment can be given depending upon the cause of excessive cortisol secretion. Surgery may be necessary if the tumour is found.

Hypothalamic Damage

The hypothalamus is the *control centre of your body* and is responsible for all automatic regulatory activities, like body temperature, sex drive, sleep, thirst, hunger, moods, release of hormones from glands, especially the pituitary gland.

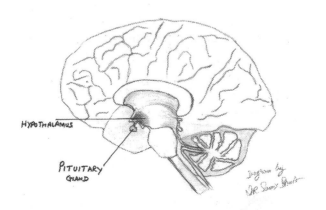

Location of our Hormone Regulators

Hypothalamic injury from any structural damage due to disease, injuries, tumour, or any kind of treatment after-effects can frequently result in the *development of obesity*. There can be a *rapid weight gain* accompanied by *severe hyperphagia* (excessive ingestion of food beyond what's needed for basic energy requirements). Weight gain occurs from the *disruption* of the normal homeostatic functioning of the *hypothalamic centres*, which are responsible for *controlling satiety and hunger* and regulating energy balance. All this might result in hyperphagia, autonomic imbalance, reduction of energy expenditure, and hyperinsulinemia.

Reducing weight is very important in these cases. Weight reduction can be possible with medications, dietary changes, and lifestyle interventions, cryolipolysis, or laser and ultrasound therapies; in extreme cases, surgery may be required.

Micronutrient Deficiencies and Mineral Toxicity

Micronutrient *deficiency* and *excess* interferes with the normal physiological functioning of the body and can be associated with a wide range of health problems, including weight gain.

People who do *yo-yo dieting* are found to be *deficient* in micronutrients, such as vitamin D, vitamin E, chromium, molybdenum, iodine, biotin, zinc, iron, and folic acid.

I have already taken up important vitamins and minerals in detail in the initial chapters.

The important thing to remember is that you should always *consult your doctor* before starting on any *fat-soluble vitamins* (like vitamin A, D, E, K) and minerals because *excess of these micronutrients* can land you into *many more medical problems* as excess of them cannot be excreted. Until and unless you are deficient in them, try not to be regular with them. Taking water-soluble vitamins, on the other hand, like B complex is a safe option because your body excretes the excessive amount of B vitamins without harm.

Vitamin overdose refers to a condition of high storage levels of vitamins, which can lead to *toxic symptoms*. Generally, toxic levels of vitamins are achieved through high supplement intake and not from dietary sources. Toxicities of fat-soluble vitamins can also be caused by a large intake of highly fortified foods. These mineral and vitamin toxicities can make your *metabolic rate sluggish* as they are toxic to the liver, so the fat-burning tendency of your body reduces, and you start *piling fat*.

B^{12} Deficiency

All pure vegetarians, vegans, and all seniors should have their B^{12} deficiency ruled out with *methylmalonic acid testing*. B^{12} deficiency can cause gait and balance problems, tremor, orthostatic hypotension, paraesthesia, confusion, and dementia in old people, and this *reduces the metabolic rate*.

Weight loss surgeries have been shown to cause lots of micronutrient deficiencies. According to scientific studies, *anaemia* was shown to develop in more than one-third of the patients. Nearly two-thirds of the patients had *reduced* levels of vitamin B^{12}. It was also observed that such patients had abnormally low levels of other fat-soluble vitamins compared to patients using non-invasive methods like ultrasound.

Prominent vitamin and mineral deficiencies were of:

- folate
- iron
- potassium.

While prompt recognition and treatment has prevented the development of a clinical deficiency syndrome in most patients, 12 per cent patients became anaemic most likely because of micronutrient deficiency related to *gastric bypass surgeries*. Thiamine deficiency—related neurologic sequelae, immune paralysis, and marrow suppression were seen in *post-surgery* trials.

Micronutrient deficiencies and anaemia made long-term frequent metabolic assessment of these patients mandatory.

A side effect of weight loss surgeries is that you die younger though thinner, so it should be your last resort if possible.

Heavy Metal Toxicity

It is fast becoming common phenomena globally.

Heavy metals are all those metals that have specific gravities five times greater than water. Examples are iron, zinc, copper, manganese, lead, mercury, arsenic, cadmium. The list is long. It has more than *thirty* elements that are in the radar of being significant to humans.

Small amounts of some of these heavy metals are actually necessary for *good health*. Examples are iron (which everyone knows about) and some other minerals like chromium, cobalt, copper, manganese, zinc. But in *large doses*, these may cause acute or chronic toxicity (*poisoning*). Heavy metal toxicity can result in damaged or reduced mental functions and central nervous function, lower energy levels, and damage to blood composition, lungs, kidneys, liver, and other vital organs. Long-term exposure may result in slowly progressing physical, muscular, and neurological degenerative processes that mimic Alzheimer's disease, Parkinson's disease, muscular dystrophy, and multiple sclerosis. Allergies are not uncommon, and repeated long-term contact with some metals or their compounds may even cause cancer.

Mercury is a metal that is directly related to weight gain. My main concern, being a weight loss expert, is mercury simply because there is a strong relation between mercury and *weight gain*. Mercury is found in elemental form, organic form as well as inorganic forms around us. Mercury continues to be used in thermometers, thermostats, and dental amalgams. Many researchers suspect dental amalgam as being a possible source of mercury toxicity (Omura et al. 1996; O'Brien 2001).

People in the mining industry and in the manufacturing of fungicides, thermometers, and thermostats are specially exposed to heavy doses of mercury.

Dental amalgam is suspected as being a possible source of mercury toxicity from chronic exposure, but the studies are not very conclusive. Dental associations throughout the world agree and support ongoing research to develop new materials that will prove to be as safe as dental amalgam. The fact is that metallic mercury used by dentists to manufacture dental amalgam is shipped as a hazardous material to a dentist's clinic. ADA (American Dentist Association) discourages the removal of existing amalgam fillings from teeth because of the toxicity risk.

The symptoms of toxicity can be overweight, anxiety, forgetfulness, emotional instability, insomnia, fatigue, weakness, anorexia, cognitive and motor dysfunction, and kidney damage.

According to the Agency for Toxic Substances and Disease Registry, *mercury levels* in the blood should not exceed *50 micrograms/litre.*

Treatment of mercury poisoning has to be very specific according to individual symptoms and signs. Your doctor will be taking detailed history of possible exposure, so be very cooperative with your doctor. Your physical examinations and treatment vary with the age, health status, amount or form of the substance that was suspected to be the culprit, and the time since exposure (absorption rate).

Supportive care (intravenous fluids, cardiac stabilization, exchange transfusion, dialysis) and decontamination (charcoal, cathartics, emesis, gastric lavage, surgery)— these procedures might require hospitalization or treatment in a healthcare centre.

Chelation therapy is used to treat heavy metal toxicity and to remove metals that accumulate in the body tissues as what happens in some genetic disorders like haemochromatosis. Chelation, decontamination procedures as well as supportive measures are used in combination. The therapies can be very complex and highly individualized, tailored to the specific needs of each individual and requiring the expertise of trained and experienced professionals, sometimes a team of professionals. Self-diagnosis and treatment is life-threatening and should never be attempted.

Genetic Factors

Bardet–Biedl Syndrome

It is a genetic disorder that produces effects on multiple body systems. It is characterized principally by *obesity*, mental retardation, hypogonadism, and renal failure in some cases.

Note: It is important to recognize that, except in *very rare cases* as mentioned above, genes that impact body weight do not directly cause obesity. Rather, genetic make-up influences the likelihood of weight gain when the person lives in an environment that supports eating calories in excess or less physical activity or both.

The genes found on **chromosome 1, 6, and 10 are found to be *faulty* in patients**. What is the exact gene? No one knows yet. In 95 per cent of the cases, genes for gaining weight cannot be researched unless the environment supports them.

The environment has a big role in weight control. I will talk about this in my next two chapters.

Bulimia Nervosa

Bulimia nervosa is an *eating disorder* in which a person *binges and then purges*. A person suffering from bulimia will *eat a lot of food at once* and then try to get rid of the food by vomiting, using *laxatives* and other medications, or sometimes even *over-exercising*!

If you eat a large amount of food within any two-hour period with the feeling that you cannot stop eating or control what or how much you are eating and all this happens at least two times in a week for three consecutive months, you are likely to be labelled as having bulimia nervosa. People with bulimia are preoccupied with their weight and body image. Bulimia is associated with depression and other psychiatric disorders.

People with bulimia may have the following signs and symptoms:

1. binge-eating of high-carbohydrate foods (secretly)
2. exercising for *hours*
3. eating until painfully full
4. going to the bathroom after meals
5. loss of control over eating with guilt and shame
6. body weight that goes up and down
7. constipation, diarrhoea, nausea, gas, abdominal pain with dehydration
8. irregular periods or lack of menstrual periods
9. damaged tooth enamel and bad breath
10. sore throat or mouth sores
11. depression.

Genes may play a part. There is some evidence that a woman who has a sister or mother with bulimia have a *higher risk* of developing this condition. Psychological factors also play an important part. Let's say that a person has low self-esteem or is not able to control impulsive behaviours and has trouble expressing anger. Some people with bulimia may have a history of sexual abuse. People with bulimia may also experience depression, self-mutilation, substance abuse, and obsessive-compulsive behaviour.

In my clinical experience, I have only two patients with bulimia nervosa. One of the females is now out of touch; she is a celebrity. And the other patient is now improving with the teamwork of her psychiatrist, me, and a dietician from our clinic. Getting rid of an eating disorder needs teamwork to help the patient.

Treatment of Bulimia

These cases are very tricky. It combines psychotherapy, family therapy, and medication. We have to reduce weight and, wherever possible, eliminate the binge-eating and purging behaviours of patients. The motivation of patients to cooperate in the restoration of healthy eating patterns and their participation in the treatment are very important. As doctors, it's our duty to provide education regarding healthy nutrition and eating patterns, treatments of associated psychiatric conditions (including mood and impulse regulation, self-esteem, and behaviour), anti-depressants, family counselling, and prevent relapse.

Even after all the efforts by the patient, doctors, and weight loss experts, many people relapse after treatment and need long-term care. Possible complications from repeated bingeing and purging include problems with the digestive system (oesophagus, stomach) ulcers, and micronutrient deficiencies. People with suicidal thoughts or severe symptoms may need to be hospitalized.

Type 1 and Type 2 Diabetes

Now here is a surprise. Treatment of diabetes is a double-edged sword as far as weight is concerned. How?

As you go through the next paragraph and the congruent picture, you will have a sense of what I mean. So let's roll.

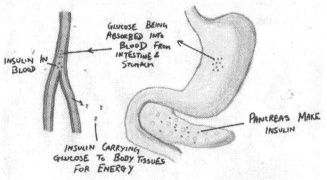

Diagram Showing Insulin's Function in body

If you have type 1 diabetes and are being treated with insulin injections, this can be one of the reasons that you are gaining weight.

In the beginning, when a person is not diagnosed with diabetes and has very high blood sugar, patients may be showing weight loss because of peeing glucose and thus losing energy and so a negative energy balance.

And when diabetes is finally diagnosed and the person is started with insulin shots, the patient often notices that she or he is gaining weight. The same thing may happen if you have type 2 diabetes and are controlling your diabetes with drugs or insulin injections.

Why Do We Start Gaining Weight When Diabetes Is in Control?

Here is an explanation for you to understand: Insulin acts like a truck that carries glucose and fats from the blood into the cells of the body so that your body can store that circulating fat and provide energy to various parts of the body by the utilization of circulating glucose. This makes sense because in the absence of insulin, both glucose and fats keep on circulating in the bloodstream and causes health concerns. Here is the mistake that God did. I call it a *transportation error.* God should have made different trucks for glucose transportation. Let's name them *sugar trucks* and, for fat transportation, *fat trucks*. This was a fundamental mistake. GOD made only one type of truck—*insulin*—for both sugar and fat *transport*, and who is suffering? Me and you. Another excuse not to lose weight. LOL.

You must understand that insulin is a hormone that delights to deposit fats in your body, especially when the doses you're taking are high. This can lead to weight gain, and that is not good to keep your diabetes under control.

While you're taking insulin, especially in high doses, you feel the need to have some snacks to avoid hypoglycaemia.

But this is not good if your snack is loaded with fat as it will result in you gaining a lot of extra weight.

The best thing to do here is to reduce the doses of insulin and to rather optimize it so that you don't have hypoglycaemia. If you find that your blood glucose levels are not optimal, you may consult your doctor to decrease the doses of insulin injected.

People with type 2 diabetes in the early stages have a condition called *insulin resistance*, and their bodies are able to make insulin but can't use it properly to move glucose into the cells. As a result, the amount of glucose in the blood rises. The pancreases have to make more insulin to try to *overcome the problem of hyperglycaemia*. Eventually, the pancreas wears out by working overtime and may no longer be able to produce enough insulin to keep blood glucose levels within a normal range. At this point, a person has type 2 diabetes.

People who don't have diabetes can still have insulin resistance. Those with insulin resistance have a higher risk of developing type 2 diabetes and are usually obese, which we technically call the *pre-diabetic stage*.

Summary

- Diseased obesity is an overweight/obesity condition caused by a *disease or pathology*. The examples are below:
  o *Hypothyroidism* is a condition in which the thyroid function becomes slow. A person may

start gaining weight, feel tired or depressed, and start having muscle pains.

o *Polycystic ovary syndrome* (PCOS) is a condition that affects the ovaries (absent or irregular periods). A person suffering from PCOS will not only gain weight but will also show acne (spotty skin), hirsutism (excessive hair growth on the face and body), difficulties getting pregnant, thinning of scalp hair.

o *Viral infection* can also be a cause of weight gain. Scientists observed that obese humans have a higher prevalence of serum neutralizing antibodies to Ad-36, the suspected virus responsible for weight gain.

o *Cushing's syndrome* is caused by an oversecretion of ACTH by the pituitary, leading to excess cortisol secretion. Symptoms like upper body obesity, rounded face, increased fat around the neck, and thinning of arms and legs are highlights of this disease.

o *Hypothalamic injury* from any structural damage due to disease, injuries, tumour, or any kind of treatment after-effects can frequently result in the development of obesity.

o *Micronutrient deficiency* interferes with the normal physiological functioning of the body and can be associated with a wide range of health problems, including weight gain.

o *Genetic disorders* can produce effects on multiple body systems. Disorders are characterized principally by obesity, mental retardation, hypogonadism, and renal failure in some cases.

o   *Bulimia nervosa* is an eating disorder in which a person binges and then purges. The affected person may eat a lot of food at once and then try to get rid of the food by vomiting, using laxatives and other medications, or sometimes even over-exercising. Weight gain may or may not be there.

o   *Diabetes* can also be one of the main causes of obesity!

Chapter 6

The reason that I made food addict obesity a separate class is that conventional methods of diet, exercise, and energy balance don't work on food addicts at all. And these are the patients I have categorized separately from other overweight/obesity categories. And I am sure all the doctors and scientists would recognize this as a separate group because the treatment protocol has to be different in these cases.

In simple terms, food addiction is a chronic disease and can be defined as *an unhealthy relationship with food*, so much so that a person is unable to stop or control food intake despite of the immense pain, suffering, and overall harm it causes.

My Technical Data

In the last seven years of my practice and after treating over 3,200 patients (most of them being from the urban population), about 30 per cent of them fall in this category. This is surprising because they are never separated from other obesity/overweight patients and almost 100 per cent food addicts are fat. Those 1,000 patients clearly fall in this category, and if I segregate it further into sexes, the female-male ratio is 3:1.

Note: Please do not confuse food addiction with bulimia nervosa, in which a person purges after eating. I am not taking bulimia here because it is a serious psychological problem in 2 to 4 per cent of the white female population. I have taken it in the category of diseased obesity, not here in food addiction obesity.

Having said that, there might be some window of error in technical data. Allow me to explain it with help of a metaphor.

My practical experience as a medical officer back in my general-practice days nine to ten years back with obese individuals (most of them from the urban population of North India) was that 20 per cent of them were in the food addiction category. The reason I believe there is a higher percentage of the food addict obese population in my present data is the weight loss clinic that we are running.

Read on, and the concept will sink in.

Now, imagine this mathematical variation: As you know, I have categorized obesity into four chunks. Just for a minute, if we assume that there are ten people who are overweight or obese (as you have read in last two chapters), let's imagine that the ratio of those ten people come out to be 6:1:2:1 (i.e. six are ignorant obese, one of them is diseased obese, two people are food addict obese, and the one that is left is knowledgemongering obese, which I will cover in the next chapter). We have all the diet and exercise knowledge freely available in the form of charts, chats, web. In real life, we get all the information through friends, family, well-wishers, advisers! So now imagine that two of the six ignorant obese did all the things through advice—exercise, diet, meditation, positive thinking, motivation—like we all do in real life and lost weight, they won't be coming to a weight loss clinic like ours. So my exposure is going to be with those eight people out of ten, who are not getting the results from advice. My data becomes 4:1:2:1. So now, in terms of percentage data, this will show more people in other categories. I hope you got the concept.

I have very less data of prevalence of obesity in rural areas as I have hardly treated 154 patients from rural backgrounds and had only six patients falling in this category of obesity, so the percentage in the rural category may vary.

My Story as a Food Addict Conqueror

This is my own real chestnut confession hidden from the limelight in this chapter.

Why did I start this weight loss journey? Was it interest, was it passion, was it money? What was it? The answer is simply complex. First, it was passion for weight loss, and then somewhere in the middle of my passionate journey, I was at the receiving end! Yep, I was an overweight food addict as well. I became a food addict and felt like a fool, a fool who knows everything about the human body's functions, about food, about supplements, about exercise, about body awareness, about sports and still couldn't control my own life. What a shame it was. What a shame. As I am rewriting this page, my eyes are wet with the thought of that person I used to be, absolutely caged and locked in food.

I would spend evenings eating non-stop, mostly breakfast cereals, then some jagerry, and then sugar-free ice cream. I had 5,000 to 7,000 calories at a time! I calculated it so many times, so many times. I used to feel so out of control that while going back home, I used to robotically park my car at a local supermarket, pick up different packets of breakfast cereals, and ate them all in one go. I use to think, How can someone stop at just 30 to 40 grams of cereals when I don't feel full even after consuming a 400-gram pack! I was absolutely freaking out.

I used to fight with my sister, who used to stop me from destroying my physique. My parents were also upset with everything, and they did whatever they could to support me. This behaviour repeated every alternate day as if someone rang a bell in my mind and I had to gather stuff from the supermarket, bring it home, and eat all of it. And I knew that I was acting like a proper a**hole towards my duties as a family member, as a doctor, as a friend. I felt like a sack of sloth.

I did everything possible to stop me—one meal a day, two meals a day, five meals a day, eight snacks a day, high protein, high carbs, high fats—but nothing worked. And when it was time, I had to eat. Whether I ate twenty-four hours before that or one hour before, it didn't matter. I studied case histories, talked to the best doctors in the world, chatted with my other physician friends all over the world and my father as well. It took me long to come out with diagnosis and treatment options for food addiction.

I knew that my life was heading towards a dead end, and I had to find a solution to it. That was the time when my perception to this category of obesity increased and helped me become a better doctor capable of envisioning the smallest details in my weight loss client's journey. You guys know that when your threshold of obesity as a disease reduces, you start seeing what normal people can't.

For me, the biggest question was, as a weight loss doctor, how would I cure myself? My earlier perception about obesity was that diet, exercise, and medicine were the only ways to good health. I got a battery of blood tests done; out of that, some tests came back positive, but those were because of the shitty processed food I was eating. I started exploring the options in my mind, whether I should go to the medical school's dietician, my teacher, a psychologist, a psychiatrist, the meditation gurus, holistic medications, Ayurveda, yoga, acupressure, massage, or to the Himalayas!

I tried a lot of things, and some of those things worked for a few days and then failed after some time, and the same food was addicting again. Enough were my grievances to inspire me to know more of what the missing link was in all the diet books, all the weight loss books, all the websites that I've gone through had failed to address—one of the important causes of weight gain in a lot of people. Now I am practising and have realized that there are so many people I can help who are suffering from it.

Ladies and gentlemen, please welcome the mighty food addiction.

Let's explore the very bases of food addition. Why do people have food addiction?

- We have always enjoyed good food in memorable times—birthdays, anniversaries, parties, and special occasions. Everything good revolves around foods. Our brain slowly starts linking high sugar, high fatty food, and alcohol with good times. On top of that, food and liquor companies, through their advertisements worth trillions, don't let you forget to link good times with all those fats, sugars, and drinks. It's all good for 70 per cent of the people to eat, pray, love, party, and carry on, but the minority, the 30 per cent, are crushed and squashed and become addicted to food or liquor or both.

- Boredom is another reason. We start hogging food to stimulate pleasure from eating. Food which brings a sense of belonging makes us feel better because we kind of run a quick memory flash of goodness in our brain. Our brain is wired to link food to good times, and when we feel good, it numbs boredom.

- A lot of people start linking sexual life with high-calorie food, like chocolates and liquor. People who are prone to become food addicts, and their sexual lives are hampered if they don't combine alcohol or high-calorie food with sex—another linkage made in your memory.

- Stress is often seen as an important reason for food addiction, as you can see in the flow chart below. I call it a love letter to addiction. After seeing my love letter, addiction may or may not want to love me back, just like a real proposal. ☺

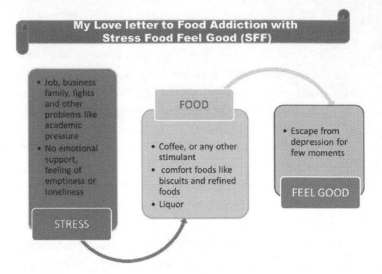

My quote for food addicts is this: 'Folks who eat for pleasure shall find that pleasure eats them.'

No one wants to be addicted to junk food, but for some of us, the experience feels good and causes the extra release of pleasure chemicals, and we want to have more food.

Question is that why only *30 per cent* becomes overweight due to food addiction?

For 70 per cent of the people, food addiction is bullshit, and they can say that because, for them, food addiction is an excuse to eat more and they are not the ones who are in deep shit called addiction.

'Excess of eating is a bad habit,' my friend told me, and my answer to him was 'I can get rid of all my habits.' I had a dentist friend who told me that everyone had a habit of brushing their teeth in a unique way, starting from one part of the mouth and finishing exactly where they started, and he said, 'You can't change it.' The very next day, I changed my habit of brushing and started brushing from the opposite side. It was a bit odd, but I did it, and even today, after a year of changing my habits, I brush with my newly acquired way. No problem there. But with food, it took me (and my well-wishers) a very painful, traumatic, courageous, and skilful long time, and it required tons of patience from the side of my family, doctors, and friends who helped me to come out of it. Just like in any chronic disease, I had to be careful about my eating.

It might be lack of willpower. My answer used to be 'Who wants to hog?' I had an awesome physique with a six-pack, and I ruined it in a matter of months. I was overweight in no time. I thought of consulting a psychiatrist. I was fortunately all right according to him.

But all my willpower to control my food consumption was there earlier. Then what happened lately when I needed it the most.

I thought maybe I am weak, but I had a lot of setbacks in life before that which could have psyched me, just like you. It is part of life, and I couldn't digest the fact that me being weak was a relevant basis to explain the problem.

Then I concluded that it was a disease that could have been missed by my diagnosis.

What is the reason for only 30 per cent of the obese population being food addicts and not others? Let's expose some predisposing factors that can trigger food addiction.

- Some studies in the 1980s have shown that if we start high-glycaemic foods early in our life, chances are that that it will be twice as hard for us to get rid of food addiction than those who did not. Children are anyways exposed to junk food early in life; that can add to the chances of them becoming food addicts.

- Unhappy families with lack of trust among couples and divorced people are likely to be the targets.

- Gays, bisexuals, and the transgender population are highly susceptible to food addiction and obesity because of lack of support from their families.

- In my practical experience, as I have shown in the beginning of this chapter, women are three times more susceptible to have food addiction than males because of their responsibilities on both the family and work fronts. On the top of all this, their spouses are physically assaulting them—even worse—and gravitation to food and being overweight just cascades from the situation, increasing the guilt and shame.

The vicious cycle goes like this:

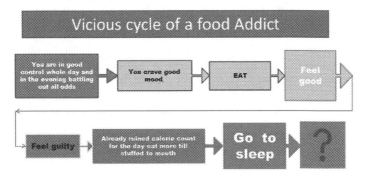

In this vicious cycle, I haven't mentioned the add-ons like advice from people on what to do and what not to. If you think that this is your pattern, go to your family doctor or weight loss clinic run by a doctor. You need proper structured help. Mere advice won't help you at all. If you can imagine read my lips, advice won't help, but proper medical help will. Let's continue with the journey.

Facts on Food Addiction

Here are some amazing facts that might put some light on the puzzle of food addiction.

To understand food addiction, I have a real story of our brain that you will always remember if you read carefully.

This is a story of our brain. Read on, and you will understand it.

The main players in the story of our brain are:

- temporal lobe
- limbic system
- anterior extreme of basal ganglia called amygdala.

There is another part of the brain that is of significance to food and that is insular cortex. Insula handles the disgust taste and nausea part. Imaging studies of a functional brain have shown that the insular cortex is activated when drug abusers are exposed to environmental cues that trigger cravings. The direct link between the insular cortex and the (mesotelencephalic) dopamine system, which forms the backbone of *dopamine reward theories of addiction*, is yet to be established.

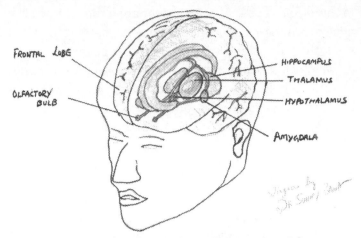

FRONTAL LOBE

OLFACTORY BULB

HIPPOCAMPUS

THALAMUS

HYPOTHALAMUS

AMYGDALA

Diagram showing Important Components Of Dopamine Reward Theory

The other prominent player in this cocktail of addiction, as I have mentioned above, is the part of the temporal lobe handling memory, awareness of smell, emotions, vision, hearing, and equilibrium.

The prefrontal lobe stores memories that record associations with food or alcohol and make neural connections. This region of brain is known as *insula*, and the surrounding gray matter allows your consciousness to sense an urge or craving to bring on extra surge of glucose into the brain.

Let's talk of less-technical stuff and simplify the story of our brain.

There are countless nerve connections in the brain, and all these connections dictate our thinking, memories, what we feel, how we react to situations, and how we act, just like the computer languages Java or Oracle can help in building complex programs in computer software. Our brain makes complex programs, forming interconnections with nerve cells.

Remember, I told you about insulin trucks in the previous chapter. Just like insulin in blood, the brain has *neurotransmitter trucks* for transporting signals. Neurotransmitter trucks carry nerve impulses between gaps in your nerve cells, carrying impulse from one nerve cell to another in a one-way fashion.

At the junction of two nerve cells, there is *a very small space* that is called a *synapse*, and I told you earlier that the road in that synapse is only one way. There are descending neurons and receiving neurons. On the descending nerve cell, there are transporters which supply message-laden *dopamine trucks* into that synapse so that dopamine can dump the message at the surface of the receiving nerve cell. These sites where dopamine delivers the message are called receptors. After dumping the messages, dopamine trucks go back to the transporter and remain in the descending neurons till they get new messages to carry through the synapse into the receptors for another cycle of transportation. The dumping of messages by dopamine at the receptor level gives us a *sense of pleasure*. There are many dopamine receptors and transporters in a single synapse, so the above-mentioned cycle of dumping of pleasure message and going back causes a chain reaction of pleasure sensations that you get.

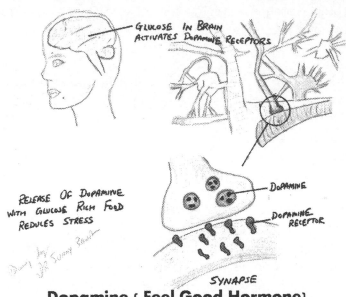

<u>Dopamine (Feel Good Hormone)</u>
<u>Relation To Food</u>

When you are happy with the food, this is what happens in your brain.

When you have sugary, buttery food, more dopamine is released, and you get that sugar high. When we feel bad because of some external situations, tension, or stress, we subconsciously want to feel better, and the easiest way is to grab that cookie or ice cream and feel good for some time. Maybe that's why we call them comfort food.

All this is normal if done occasionally, but things start getting dirty and abnormal when you start abusing this body mechanism every time you have a situation. Every time you are stressed, your brain makes memory connections. To release that tension, you have to have high-calorie food, which will release pleasure chemicals and numb your everyday problems. This same mechanism works with alcoholics. The same pleasure chemicals are released, and you feel better. So it's good that we all need pleasure in our lives, and if we know that food and alcohol can give that, why not have it?

But your brain is a supercomputer and more intelligent than you are. The brain starts developing tolerance to stimulants like food and alcohol. Every time you use these as drugs to cope up with your daily problems, the brain increases the threshold, and the same amount of alcohol or food will not numb your problem in the same way it used to a few weeks back. So you start increasing the dose of comfort food to get the similar response of pleasure because an instant surge of dopamine with food fades the tension for at least some time so that you can sleep properly. That's a shortcut, my friend. Always remember that *shortcuts cut your life short*. Whoa, another quote just jumped out of my mind.

You start becoming overweight and then obese, and you start getting other chronic diseases.

And not only this. As they say, *a high comes with a low*. As your brain increases the threshold of pleasure chemicals, things that used to give you pleasure don't feel as pleasurable, causing panic attacks, making you blunt to emotions. People around you will start noticing and say. 'Don't you see that you are spoiling your health?' or 'Can't you exercise? That will elevate your mood. Don't you care about your family?' The answer is 'No, I can't because I am a food addict.' It is food that's making you blunt to the outside world.

Comfort food in tons will just release enough dopamine to keep you going. A small bite of pastry feels like a joke to a food addict because a half-kilogram cake will release the same amount of dopamine as a piece of cake to a normal person. Then we wonder why a few months back a small amount of comfort food used to be satisfying enough but now a ton of food does the same. It's because our brain has become tolerant. The name of the game is tolerance.

If you fall in the food addict obese category, which (according to my practical experience) is 30 per cent of the obese population in North India, then you don't need a fitness expert but your doctor or a certified dietician, who will know that you need a proper long-term treatment and rehabilitation, just like with any other chronic disease. And if you follow the medications given by doctors (who might want to refer you to specialized weight loss doctors or psychologists or psychiatrists for medical treatment), go by their programs, and follow their advise, things will start getting better.

How Can You Help a Family Member or a Friend Who Is Suffering from Food Addiction?

If you are worried about your friend's eating behaviour or attitude, it is important to express your concern in a loving and supportive way. It is also necessary to discuss your worries early on rather than waiting until your friend has endured many of the damaging physical and emotional effects of eating disorders. In a private and relaxed setting, talk to your friend in a calm and caring way about the specific things you have seen or felt that have caused you to worry.

What to Say Step by Step

1. *Set a time to talk.* Set aside a time for a private, respectful meeting with your friend or family member to discuss your concerns openly and honestly in a caring, supportive way. Make sure you find some place away from other distractions.
2. *Communicate your concerns.* Share your memories of specific times when you felt concerned about his or her eating or exercise behaviours. Explain that you think these things may indicate that there could be a problem that needs professional attention.
3. *Ask the affected friend to explore these concerns* with a counsellor, doctor, nutritionist, or other health professional who is knowledgeable about eating issues. If you feel comfortable doing so, offer to help your friend make an appointment or accompany her or him on their first visit.
4. *Avoid conflicts or a battle of the wills* with them. If she or he refuses to acknowledge that there is a problem or any reason for you to be concerned, restate your feelings and the reasons for them, and leave yourself open and available as a supportive listener.
5. *Avoid placing shame, blame, or guilt* on her or him regarding their actions or attitudes. Do not use accusatory *you* statements like 'You are acting irresponsibly'. Instead, use *I* statements. For example, 'I'm concerned about you because you

had much more than normal food' or 'It makes me afraid to see you eat'.

6. *Avoid giving simple solutions*—for example, 'If you'd just stop, then everything would be fine!'

7. *Express your continued support.* Remind him or her that you care and want him or her to be healthy and happy.

After talking with them, if you are still concerned with their health and safety, find a medical professional to talk to. This is probably a challenging time for all of you. It could be helpful for you as well as the person suffering from food addiction to discuss your concerns and seek assistance and support from a professional.

Treatment

Treatment includes individual, group, or family therapy and medical management and support by a doctor. Support groups, nutrition counselling, and psychiatric medications under careful medical supervision have also proven helpful for some individuals.

Some medications have been shown to be helpful. Ideally, whatever treatment offered should be tailored to the individual, and this will vary according to both the severity of the disorder and the patient's individual problems, needs, and strengths.

Typically, care is provided by a licensed health professional, including but not limited to a psychologist, psychiatrist, social worker, nutritionist, and/or family doctor.

Care should be coordinated and provided by a health professional with the expertise and experience in dealing with eating-related problems.

Treatment must address the eating disorder symptoms as well as the psychological, biological, interpersonal, and cultural forces that contribute or maintain the eating disorder. Nutritional counselling is also necessary and should incorporate education about nutritional needs and planning for and monitoring rational choices of the individual patient.

Warning: Self-medication in these cases can be dangerous and can induce suicidal symptoms in patients, so please seek a doctor's help. The exact treatment needs of each individual will vary. It is important for individuals struggling with an eating disorder to find a health professional they trust to help coordinate and oversee their care.

Summary

- *Food addiction* is a chronic disease and can be defined as an unhealthy relationship with food, so much so that a person is unable to stop or control food intake despite the immense pain, suffering, and overall harm it is causing.
- Around 30 per cent of my patients fall in this category of obesity. Formally, it has never been separated by other weight gain causes until and unless someone had severe psychological problems like bulimia nervosa.

- The primary neurotransmitter of the reward pathway is dopamine, which explains why we get food addiction. Although food addiction involves various locations in the brain reward system, they share a final common action in that they increase dopamine levels in the brain reward system and thus addiction.

- It is also necessary to discuss your worries early on rather than waiting until your family member or friend who might be suffering from food addiction has endured many of the damaging physical and emotional effects of eating disorders. In a private and relaxed setting, talk to your friend in a calm and caring way about the specific things you have seen or felt that have caused you to worry.

- Treatment includes individual, group, or family therapy and medical management and support by a doctor. Support groups, nutrition counselling, weight loss clinics, and psychiatric medications under careful medical supervision have also proven helpful for some individuals.

Chapter 7

Knowledgemongering Obese

The father of medicine, Hippocrates, said once, '**There are in fact two things, science and opinion; the former begets knowledge, the latter ignorance.'**

I have separated those opinion-based ignorant obese as a special case of obesity where treatment is based on building trust as knowledgemongers don't trust anyone. They will google everything you say, and they don't trust anyone, so they remain obese. I call them Mister or Miss Know-It-All.

I have a fair number of knowledgemongering obese clients in my clinical set-up, and I am sure doctors of all the streams must be having similar experiences like I am having; in fact, doctors, therapists, dieticians, and weight loss experts whom I personally know agree that they have knowledgemongers in their clinical practices. In my clinical practice, knowledgemonger obesity is as high as 20 per cent of the total obese population.

In my definition, a person who creates hindrance in the execution of his or her own therapy by implementing their own fundamentals derived from unreliable resources in weight loss therapy. The resources they access can be based on their little knowledge, through the Net, through their own old experiences, advise from people without the knowledge of a doctor, dietician, or fitness expert who can treat them for weight loss.

The only difference between the ignorant obese and knowledgemongering obese is that the ignorant obese have a tendency of high degree of trust, and they cooperate with doctors and therapists fully in their treatment plans. Of course, they have a number of queries, but they stick to the plan given by the health practitioner. They do not make their own plans, and they stick to the plan to the Z rather than do their own stuff. In a practical setting, you have to treat knowledgemongers as a separate category requiring different protocol; otherwise, they won't get results because they won't stick to any protocol.

In the obese/overweight urban population, their percentage is only 5 per cent, and I expect it to increase over time. So I have categorized them separately as they have very high chances of discontinuing therapy and are one of the most difficult patients to treat.

Symptoms and Signs of Knowledgemongering Obese

I have identified two types of knowledgemongering obese.

1. **Type A**
   This is a person who goes to a physician or a weight loss expert and have already tried a lot of diets and

programs that they have little hope of getting any benefit from experts. It is very difficult to treat these patients because they lose trust in themselves and they don't trust physicians, therapists, dieticians, and whoever is trying to help them. Many of my patients have tried going to the gym, dance classes, all kinds of diets, yoga, spa therapies, diet pills, liposuction—almost everything! In case of the knowledgemongering obese, it's the doctor who has to be patient and do whatever she or he can do to help them and build trust. Once they start getting results, the trust level increases.

2. **Type B**

   In my clinical practice, 2 per cent of the cases qualify as knowledgemongering obese. Recognizing them is very simple. In the very first appointment, if they have a battery of test questions (not queries—I am sure doctors and patients know the difference between a query and a test), testing the doctor's general knowledge. If a physician does a detailed counselling—of course, on weight gain with patience—they will find that knowledgemongering obese (type B) have superficial knowledge about so many things and that their history will reveal the list of supplements and vitamins and minerals they took to lose weight. They will tell the doctor their detailed knowledge about supplements with background studies done on those supplements, justifying the reason to take so many more supplements.

> Treating them mean giving them clear instructions about the protocol of weight loss and telling them to stop all the nutrition supplements and to take the vitamins as instructed by the doctor.

I have very few cases from this category of patients.

I remember one of my patients who was taking whey protein along with a 2,000-calorie non-vegetarian diet. He was doing weight training, and the battery of supplements he had taken in the past one year had no resultant weight loss. He took ginseng, hydroxycitric acid, L-carnitine, psyllium, pyruvate, St John's wort, and caffeine capsules. We as physicians should caution patients about the use of these supplements and closely monitor those who choose to use these products. I had to tell him to stop everything. Even the whey protein was not needed as he was eating ten eggs in a day and 100 grams of roasted chicken at night. Sometimes overnutrition with supplements can become a major cause of gaining weight.

Lab Tests have shown that protein uptake of the body after having starchy food is negligible in obese as compared to lean people. In lean people, blood protein levels reduce rapidly. The takeaway message from these studies is that the need for extra protein supplements is more in lean people, like your trainer, who might need quick proteins after workout. But for you, it's overnutrition, just adding fat to your already bulging body.

A controlled study done in the Department of Brain and Cognitive Sciences, Massachusetts Institute of Technology, Cambridge, showed that obese/overweight people have much, much higher blood levels of the branched-chain amino acids (simple proteins), phenylalanine, and tyrosine and that the levels of these amino acids reduced very less in response to carbohydrate intake as compared to lean controls, who had reported a fall in blood BCAA. An overweight person never runs out of protein pool in the blood, so extra protein in the form of supplement might act as overnutrition and add to your weight.

The molecular dynamics of obese and lean people are different. What works on a lean individual may not work on the obese because of a number of factors. I believe one must always seek professional help before starting supplements.

There is no harm in asking your doctor before you start any supplement (except for a multivitamin pill), and your doctor would be the best judge. As it's said, **'Everything in excess is opposed to nature and its harmony'.**

Is 'Whey' Protein Powder Making Me Fat?

One of our newly joined patient (who is taking whey protein after workouts) asked me this question. Someone told her that she would lose weight with whey in water, but the fact of the matter is that she was gaining weight faster than earlier when she was not on whey!

I told her two reasons for her shocking weight gain:

- There is increase in muscle bulk. (Yes, females also gain muscles. I'll discuss this hot topic tomorrow. LOL.)
- The other reason of her gaining fat was because the total number of calories had increased.

Promptly she asked me another question, 'I have heard that eating dietary fat and simple sugars make you fat, but you are saying that even proteins and complex carbs increase body fat if taken in excess. Why is it so?'

Yes, she was right. Excess of fat and simple sugars in the diet increases the maximum amount of body fat, but at the end of the day, it's the excess amount of calories that makes you fat. And for your body, it doesn't matter where those calories come from—proteins, carbohydrates, or fats. Pick any of these in excess, and they will all convert into fat! (An exception to this rule is if you have any medical problem; in that case, even water will make you fat!)

Some interesting facts you didn't know about your body

Your body is a remarkable piece of art, a supercomputer, and a super chemical reaction laboratory. In your body, carbohydrates, proteins, and fats can all be formed from any of the three. Before you react to this comment, remember the terms *non-essential fats*, *non-essential proteins*. What does *non-essential* mean?

You will say, 'Oh, that's simple, they are not essential.' And I will say, 'Yes, they are not essential because your body can make them by converting proteins, carbohydrates, and fats into one another.' Yes, my friend, your body is already packed with enzymes and chemicals to form any of the three from any one macronutrient.

If you are really serious about weight loss, then eat a balanced meal with proteins, fats, and carbohydrates. Nothing is fatty if you consume it in moderation; rather, your body needs all of them in the right proportions to function normally.

Takeaway message

Proteins can make you fat when you eat too much protein. Protein cannot be stored for energy; the body converts it to other compounds, like fatty acids and carbohydrates. This means that when you eat more protein than your body needs, it gets stored as *body fat*.

Eat good. Live good.

Summary

- A person who creates hindrance in the execution of his or her own therapy to lose weight by implementing their own fundamentals derived from unreliable resources, leading to disappointment in reaching their desired weight goals, are knowledgemongering obese.

- It is very difficult to treat these patients because they lose trust in themselves. They don't trust physician, therapist, dietician, and whoever is trying to help them lose weight because, according to them, they have tried it all but nothing has worked on them.

- Another type of knowledgemongers have superficial knowledge about so many things. Their history will reveal a battery of supplements and vitamins and minerals they took for losing weight, and they have a strong justification for taking so many supplements.

- Treating them mean giving them clear instructions about the protocol of weight loss and telling them to stop all the nutrition supplements and to take the vitamins as instructed by the doctor. And once they start getting the desired results, trust starts building, and they will stick to the weight loss programme for longer times.

Chapter 8

How Can the Medical Field Help You Lose Weight?

Before I say goodbye to you till next book, I would like you to go through some medical options that your weight loss experts and doctors will have for you, depending on your lifestyle, physical examination, and blood tests.

Some Medicines That Can Help You Lose Weight

You should only use these medicines as part of a programme that includes diet, physical activity, and weight loss protocol.

Weight loss medicines may be suitable for adults who are obese, not overweight. In India physicians prescribe medicines to people having BMI above 27, and people with BMI above 25, who are associated with the risk of heart disease and other health conditions, also may benefit from these medicines.

- orlistat
  This medicine comes with strengths of 120 milligrams and 60 milligrams in capsule form.

In some countries, it is sold as OTC (over-the-counter drug), but in countries like India, you need a doctor's prescription for the same. You are required to take them with major meals. Orlistat is the only FDA-approved weight loss medicine after they banned sibutramine from the market in 2010. In fact, sibutramine is now banned all over the world. Coming back to orlistat, I have seen relatively mild weight loss effects with this drug in clinical practice. Usually, patients can expect weight loss of 1–2 kilograms in a month without much change in diet. Stagnation in losing weight or plateau usually comes in four to five months' time. There are some minor side effects with this drug I noticed in some of my patients, like oily and greasy stools. In case side effects are uncomfortable, your doctor will review the dosage. I recommend a cycle of five days on and two days off for this drug, which prevents fat-soluble-vitamin deficiencies that might occur if the drug is taken in the long term.

Sometimes a doctor will want to prescribe some fat-soluble-vitamin pills as an adjuvant to the therapy. Always ask your doctor before starting any medications. Your doctor might want some blood tests, some physical examinations, anthropometric measurements, etc. before starting off with therapy.

- sibutramine (now banned all over the world)
  This was one of the most exciting drugs in my weight loss career. I am going to reveal the ugly side of this drug in the paragraphs below.

Sibutramine is a noradrenaline and serotonin (5-HT) reuptake inhibitor drug that had an indication for treatment of obesity by primarily increasing satiety with some thermogenic effects. It was a very good drug. I have used it extensively for a good five years (2006–10), and it was effective at that. Some of my patients had shown really good results with it. It was actually one of the favourite drugs of endocrinologists throughout the world.

I still remember that year of 2010 when I had prescribed it to seven of my forty-five patients undergoing a weight loss programme that time. And I got a circular from the Ministry of Health and Family Welfare to inform us about the ban imposed on sibutramine and its formulations for human use. I was worried because those seven patients were on that drug, and I knew that if in the middle of the treatment I would stop their weight loss drug, their weight might start fluctuating, which inevitably would have a negative impact on a patient's motivation. Six patients out of seven did well and completed their weight loss programme without sibutramine. One was stuck, and our whole staff did a lot of extra efforts to motivate that man to complete his programme.

But the real twist in the story starts a few days after the ban of this drug. I was flooded with appointments, and our weight loss centre was jam-packed. Obviously, our whole staff was figuring out this phenomenon. What happened to everyone? Why was everyone in the area heading to NidSun?

Me and my sister figured it out as the 'sibutramin effect'. All the patients were on sibutramin, most of them self-prescribed, and were in panic.

That was the time I understood the gravity of the situation. People were getting that medicine from pharmacists without asking physicians, and let me tell you that it was a very dangerous drug with life-threatening side effects. Even we used to do battery of tests, ECG, individual counselling, and physical check-ups before we could prescribe it to patients, but here in our area, every obese was taking it. That was shocking to me, and I thought in my mind, *It's good that the drug is banned.* It was killing many people in many ways.

That was the time when I came out with the idea of a new class of obese, the knowledgemongering obese, those 'little knowledge is dangerous' people, and we took some drastic steps in weight loss protocol for this category of obesity.

- metformin
  Medicines to treat diabetes may cause small amounts of weight loss in people who have obesity and diabetes. It's not known how this medicine causes weight loss, but it has been shown to reduce hunger and food intake and thus help reduce the total number of calories consumed.

- fluoxetine (an SSRI)
  Fluoxetine is a medicine to treat depression. Some medicines for depression cause an initial weight

loss, and then there is a regain of weight while taking the medicine.

- topiramate and zonisamide
  These are medicines for treating seizures. These two medicines used for seizures have been shown to cause weight loss. These medicines are being studied to see whether they will be useful in treating obesity.

These are drugs that are available at your nearby health store, claiming to reduce weight:

- ephedra (now banned in many countries)
  It comes from plants and has been sold as a dietary supplement and fat burner in gyms around the world. The active ingredient in the plant is called ephedrine. Ephedrine releases noradrenaline in the brain which raises the metabolic rate and body temperature. It can exacerbate panic attacks, insomnia, and anxiety. It is not safe in high doses or for those with a heart condition, resulting in many deaths. Ephedra can cause short-term weight loss, but it also has serious side effects. In 2004, the FDA banned the sale of dietary supplements containing ephedra because of those side effects. This is a highly addictive drug.

- chromium
  Chromium is a mineral that's sold as a dietary supplement to reduce body fat. It's known to stabilize blood sugar by increasing cell sensitivity to insulin. This prevents excess blood sugar from being turned into body fat. It is very useful for some

diabetics in preventing the need for insulin. While studies haven't found any weight loss benefit from chromium, there are a few serious side effects from taking it in high doses.

- fibre
  Guar gum, chitosan, and psyllium have been shown to cause at least a half-kilogram-a-week reduction in weight when taken at about 5 grams before each meal, but they have not been evaluated, and excesses will cause a lot of bloating and vitamin deficiencies.

- diuretics and herbal laxatives
  These products cause you to lose water weight, not fat. They also can lower your body's potassium levels, which may cause heart and muscle problems.

- hoodia
  Hoodia is a cactus that's native to Africa. It's sold in pill form as an appetite suppressant. However, no firm evidence shows that hoodia works. No large-scale research has been done on humans to show whether hoodia is effective or safe.

- bromelaine
  It is also known to help lose weight, but again, when controlled studies are done, there are no concrete effects.

- CLA
  At the Department of Human Nutrition's Center for Advanced Food Studies at the Royal Veterinary and Agricultural University, DK-1958 Frederiksberg

C. in Denmark did a study on CLA, and the results were that CLA appears to attenuate increases in body weight and body fat in several animal models. CLA isomers sold as dietary supplements are not effective as weight loss agents in humans and may actually have adverse effects on human health, but still you will find CLA in every other weight loss supplement. I have used this supplement in my clinical practice but got no favourable results.

- hydroxycitric acid
  Found in the herb garcinia cambogia, this inhibits fat production in animals and may also decrease appetite and is also known to reduce carbohydrate absorption. It hasn't proved its mettle yet in any lab test.

- caffeine capsules
  Caffeine is known to boost your metabolism and increase the fat-burning mechanism. You can try it or just have some black coffee before exercising to get the best results.

My friends, there are hundreds of weight loss supplements that I can write a separate book on them, but my practical experience shows little beneficial effects from any of them or maybe the patients who failed with these supplements came to me.

Future medicines that are showing some results on paper are:

- adiponectin
  It is secreted from adipose tissue into the bloodstream and is quite abundant in plasma in

relation to many other hormones. Adiponectin promotes insulin sensitivity and the survival of pancreatic β cells. Just like leptin, adiponectin acts in the brain to mediate weight loss. However, it has yet to enter clinical trials.

- combination therapy with pramlintide and leptin
  Lab trials are going on showing some promising results in overweight and obese patients with the co-administration of pramlintide and leptin by subcutaneous injection twice daily; it produced approximately 13 kilograms of weight loss, while monotherapy with either agent only resulted in approximately 8 kilograms of loss. Importantly, patients on combination therapy continued to lose weight, while those on monotherapy achieved a plateau over the duration of the study.

- oleoyl-estrone
  Oleoyl-estrone (OE) is packaged in lipoproteins derived from adipose tissue for secretion in the circulation. Like leptin, OE levels are associated with adiposity, but in contrast to leptin, obese patients exhibit reduced circulating OE. OE induces dose-dependent decreases in appetite and weight.

  In humans, oral OE (150–300 micromole/day) administered to morbidly obese patients over ten consecutive twenty-one-day trial periods followed by two-month recovery periods induced a weight loss of 38.5 kilograms over twenty-seven months. While this data was promising, subsequent randomized clinical trials failed to demonstrate significant placebo-adjusted weight loss in obese patients.

Non-Surgical Weight Loss Treatment Options

Ultrasound and Radio Frequency

This treatment is non-invasive. No anaesthesia is needed as treatment is virtually painless. And with thirty minutes of therapy session, you can see the results almost immediately with a 2-centimetre reduction in the area treated after one session. This uses acoustic waves to rupture fat cell membranes, allowing the liquefied fat to be excreted and metabolized naturally and safely from the body, just as it would metabolize fatty meals.

Patients with round tummies, love handles, buttocks, hips, and saddlebags on thighs are ideal targets for this technology. Patients usually just feel a warm, perhaps tingly sensation, or may not feel anything as the transducer is gently smoothed across the targeted area. The procedure will feel familiar to anyone who has had an ultrasound scan during pregnancy or other medical conditions.

We are using this treatment at our facility, and I have observed that fat reduction in the problem area is better handled with this weight loss therapy than by just doing physical activity. However, if a patient needs massive 20 to 30 kilograms of weight loss, we have to use it as an adjuvant therapy with proper diet, activity, behavioural therapy, and rehabilitation therapies combined with this. There are many patients who don't even qualify for this therapy, so a patient's medical history and physical examination for fat distribution is important before starting this therapy.

After treatment, patients can resume all normal activities but are instructed to eat a low-fat, low-carbohydrate diet for a few days because the body is already 'mobilizing the fat'.

Each session for one area takes about thirty minutes. The number of sessions depends on the requirement and condition of the patient for each area treated.

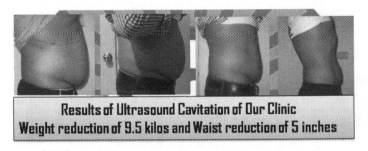

Results of Ultrasound Cavitation of Our Clinic
Weight reduction of 9.5 kilos and Waist reduction of 5 inches

Ultrasound cavitation is an effective non-surgical treatment for fat cell reduction. The procedure relies on ultrasound technology to target a patient's subcutaneous layer of the skin where fat cells are stored. Ultrasound emits sound waves to create cavitation microbubbles in the interstitial fluid. The fluid then discharges a vapour that collapses the fat cell, releasing fatty acids that are then metabolized and eliminated from the body.

Mesotherapy: A Non-Surgical Cosmetic Treatment

My few friends are doing mesotherapy for fat blasting. Mesotherapy is a medical invasive technique devised in the 1950s by Dr Michel Pistor. It is now used worldwide as a cosmetic treatment for ageing skin and to spot fat reduction. Mesotherapy involves the injection of specially prepared mixture of vitamins, amino acids, and medications into the middle layer of the skin. With this, the essential nutrients for the skin are directly injected into the areas which need treating. Target adipose fat cells are marked and injected with drugs to induce lipolysis and fat blasting; however, if a patient needs weight loss, we have to use it as an adjuvant therapy with ultrasound therapy, proper diet, activity, behavioural therapy, and rehabilitation therapies combined with this.

Cryotherapy

(Cryolipolysis's unique technology uses controlled cooling to freeze and eliminate unwanted fat cells without surgery or downtime. The procedure is FDA-cleared, safe, and effective. The results are lasting and undeniable. Cryolipolysis is a medical treatment used to destroy fat cells. Its principle relies on controlled cooling to near sub-zero temperatures for non-invasive localized reduction of fat deposits in order to reshape body contours. The exposure to cooling is set so that it causes cell death of subcutaneous fat tissue without apparent damage to the overlying skin. The procedure is billed as a non-surgical alternative to liposuction. *Cryolipolysis* is a portmanteau of *cryogenic* and *lipolysis*. Generically, the process can also be known as fat freezing.

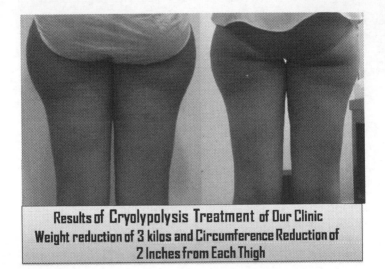

Results of Cryolypolysis Treatment of Our Clinic Weight reduction of 3 kilos and Circumference Reduction of 2 Inches from Each Thigh

The idea that cold can selectively affect fat led to the innovative cooling process developed by scientists of Harvard Medical School. Cryolipolysis technology safely delivers precisely controlled cooling to gently and effectively target the fat cells underneath the skin. The treated fat cells are crystallized (frozen), then die. Over time, your body naturally processes the fat and eliminates these dead cells, leaving a more sculpted you.

In the weeks and months to follow, your body naturally processes and eliminates the treated fat cells. Once the fat cells are gone, they're gone for good.

Laser Lipolysis

Laser lipolysis is a system that uses low-level lasers for cellulite smoothing, fat reduction, and body-shaping treatments. The treatment uses photobiomodulation to stimulate the body's natural process for releasing stored content in the adipose cells. Every day, the human body is storing excess calories from our diet in the adipose tissue. We cannot control our fat metabolism in specific areas; our body decides it. You can compare the adipose cells to a rechargeable battery, sometimes used and sometimes stored up depending on the diet and exercise. Laser lipolysis is used to trigger the release of the contents without exercise and is able to target the precise stubborn areas. Laser lipolysis is non-invasive with no pain, no needles, and no downtime.

Why? Laser lipolysis is a very good alternative for someone struggling with cellulite and stubborn fat on those problem areas. Unlike surgery and other non-surgical treatments, this is a non-contact laser treatment which involves no needles, no heat, and not even gel massage. All you need to do is sit back with laser pads on your problem areas, close your eyes, and relax. It's easy.

The laser lipolysis system has many advantages over other similar systems.

Here are just a few!

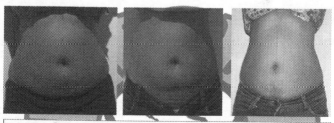

Results of Mixed Laser & Cryolypolysis Treatment of Our Clinic
Weight reduction of 5.5 kilos and Waist Circumference of 5 inches.

Independent clinical studies have shown laser lipolysis to be, in some cases, comparable to results achieved by liposuction. Ultrasound imagery shows up to 30 per cent reduction in the fat layer depth after just one treatment. Additional treatments improve results further. Results can be seen immediately after each treatment as the fat cell contents are released. Light exercise post treatment can accelerate the removal of the released fat.

By positioning the laser pads on the target areas (such as chin, upper arms, abdomen, or thighs), fat can be broken down and removed specifically from that area. This is a big advantage over diet and exercise which can reduce overall body fat but not shape individual areas.

Surgical Weight Loss

People who have extreme obesity (BMI of 40 or more) when other treatments have failed are the ones who qualify for surgical interventions. Surgery is usually the last resort that we have, especially if a person has other uncontrolled chronic conditions associated with obesity, like type 2 diabetes or heart diseases.

There are many surgical procedures, like jaw wiring, banded gastroplasty, liposuction, and Roux-en-Y gastric bypass.

- jaw wiring
  It is an operative procedure that involves wiring of your jaws so that you can limit the solid-food intake. This technique has shown promising results in the short term, but in the long term, it is less practical because of social constraints.

- banded gastroplasty
A band or staples are used to create a small pouch at the top of your stomach. This surgery limits the amount of food and liquids the stomach can hold.

- liposuction
It is a surgery using ultrasound procedure first to melt the fat and then suck it out through suction cannula. I have found similar results with non-invasive ultrasound therapies that we use in our clinic.

- Roux-en-Y gastric bypass
A small stomach pouch is created with a bypass around part of the small intestines, where most of the calories you eat are absorbed. This surgery limits food intake and reduces the calories your body absorbs.

Weight loss surgery can improve your health and weight. However, the surgery can be risky, depending on your overall health. Gastroplasty has a few long-term side effects, but you must limit your food intake dramatically anyways.

Roux-en-Y gastric bypass has more side effects (e.g. *dumping syndrome*). Nutritional deficiencies after a gastric bypass surgery for morbid obesity often cannot be prevented by standard multivitamin supplementation, a study done by the Division of Endocrinology, Dialectology, and Metabolism and the Department of Visceral Surgery (Centre Hospitalier Universitaire Vaudois, Lausanne, Switzerland) concluded. They did this study on 137 morbidly obese patients (110 women and 27 men), and 34 per cent of these patients required at least one specific supplement in addition to the multivitamin preparation. Specific supplements had been prescribed for each patient, including vitamin B^{12}, iron, calcium plus vitamin D, and folic acid, which they had to take for life!

The conclusion was that nutritional deficiencies are very common after RYGBP and can occur despite supplementation with the standard multivitamin preparation. Therefore, careful post-operative follow-up is indicated to detect and treat those deficiencies.

Gastroplasty has a few long-term side effects, and you must limit your food intake dramatically.

Liposuction has immediate side effects, but long-term side effects are less.

General side effects like wound infection, septicaemia, and hernias, especially in bypass, can occur and are no different than any normal surgical procedures.

Scientists throughout the world are worried and are doing all they can to stop this obesity epidemic, and I hope that this book will enlighten you with some facts about being obese and empower you to take good decisions to control this epidemic for your better health and fitness.

Summary

- Weight loss medicines may be suitable for adults who are obese, not overweight. Some are prescription medicines, and others are available at health stores.

- With the advent of new technologies, non-invasive procedures are fast becoming popular modes of weight loss. Of them, the prominent procedures are ultrasound weight loss procedures, radiofrequency procedures, laser lipolysis, cryotherapy, and mesotherapy.
- Invasive procedures are usually confined to morbidly obese patients on whom all other procedures have failed as these have lots of side effects and the benefits certainly weigh heavily against the risks that are involved in surgical procedures.

Chapter 9

Biochemistry Quotient

Welcome to the first step to understanding the complex world of weight loss. According to me, this is the first step to the rocket science of weight loss, so keep your energy levels up and your concentration to 100 per cent if you want to understand something profound in your life.

This is a difficult chapter to grasp, especially for a person with no medical background; basically, this chapter would be easy to understand for doctors and scientists who have clinical experience in any field of medicine. It's my own discovery by experiencing and way of putting problems in prospective and segmenting the clinical experience for taking things apart. Based on the NidSun team's clinical experiences and compiled data of almost 3,200 patients in a span of 7 years in the weight loss field, we came up with a unique name to our observations, which I call the biochemistry quotient (bio Q).

For simplifying the things, I have kept 100 as the standard value for bio Q, which should be considered as an average for the population. So when you have a bio Q of 120, you will be understood as above average, and a bio Q of below 100 is below average. Our study is based on 85 per cent North Indian patients. My guess is, this is a universal phenomenon which can only be confirmed by some controlled studies in future time to come, and I would love to have inputs from my fellow doctors and scientists all over the world to confirm the pattern.

I'll recommend that the doctor readers should be a bit imaginative and keep their critical mind on hold while they read this chapter for a better understanding of our point of view. By the end of this chapter, you will start relating to the picture that I want to portray. Remember that *a philosophy that can be proven clinically is science*!

I have used medical knowledge of perceived signs and symptoms related to specific biochemistry parameter as you go through the chapter. Before that, I would like you to know what biochemistry quotient is.

What Is Biochemistry Quotient?

Biochemistry quotient (bio Q) can be defined as the perceived ability of our body to detect various biochemistry measurements in plasma.

The detection of biochemical abnormalities by a person through perceiving signs and symptoms of a particular abnormality in blood tests is our basis for determining bio Q. Bear with me till you read the first biochemical marker that I have identified, and you will understand the concept.

Once you understand the concept and you start using it in a systematic way, you will be able to set customized treatments to individual patients and will be able to give him or her a specialized weight loss plan. Going according to bio Q actually works better then generalizing the weight loss planning.

As you already know, *biochemistry is the chemistry of life.* In length, *it's the information flow through biochemical signalling and the flow of chemical energy through metabolism; biochemical processes give rise to the incredible complexity of life.* Human biochemistry deals with the structures and functions of cellular components, such as proteins, carbohydrates, lipids, nucleic acids, and other biomolecules.

I just want to quickly remind you of biochemistry tests that we normally recommend, depending on the signs and symptoms of patients. They are alphabetically as follows:

- acetone (serum quantitative)
- acetone (urine qualitative)
- acid phosphatase (prostatic)
- acid phosphatase (total)
- adenosine deaminase
- alanine aminotransferase or ALT (SGPT)
- albumin, albumin–globulin ratio
- alkaline phosphatase
- ammonia
- amylase
- aspartate aminotransferase or AST (SGOT)
- bilirubin (total direct indirect)
- blood urea nitrogen (BUN)
- calcium
- chloride
- CK-MB, CK-NAC

- cortisol
- creatinine, creatinine with clearance of twenty-four hours
- electrolytes
- gamma glutamyl transferase (GGT)
- globulin
- glucose (fasting, postprandial, and random)
- glucose tolerance test
- lactate dehydrogenase
- lipid profile
- Mantoux test
- microalbumin (urine)
- phosphorous
- potassium
- prostate specific antigen
- protein (total)
- protein electrophoresis
- troponin I
- uric acid and more.

Other than this long list of boring tests, we at our weight loss clinic do some other tests relevant for weight loss management which I think are really important, and they are Hb, ferritin, WBC and ESR, serology (where we do C-reactive protein), clinical pathology tests (like urinalysis), TSH, T3, T4, and electrocardiogram; these are other important tests we do.

All our patients who come for weight loss have to undergo the standard operative procedure of undergoing a blood test and a urinalysis based on their clinical history. And because we have routine tests for every patient we treat, these are the things that we discovered in the last seven years.

For overweight people, my main criteria for the biochemistry quotient (bio Q) are based on six parameters, which I have illustrated in the points below. I am sure a lot of intelligent doctors out there will improvise on my concept of the *bio Q* criteria even further and use it in various fields of chronic diseases other than obesity.

First Criterion: Blood Sugar Bio Q

The normal range for FBS is 65 to 100 milligrams/decilitre, and the value of anything between 101 to 125 milligrams/decilitre is considered as borderline or, scientifically, glucose intolerance.

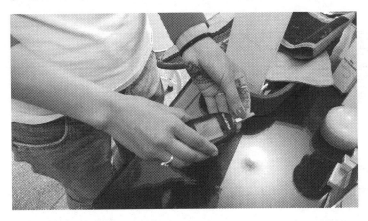

There are many patients who can perceive variations in blood sugar very well.

Now let me give you a practical example of a condition like hyperglycaemia.

My interest was in the signs and symptoms of hyperglycaemia perceived by my patients at different blood glucose levels, which is the basis of my bio Q theory, and this is an interesting finding from about 536 diabetic patients we have treated. We saw that around 7 per cent of the patients showed actual physically perceived symptoms, like tingling sensations in the legs or numbness, at blood sugar levels of as low as 130 milligrams/decilitre. And on the other side of the spectrum were 25 per cent of the patients, who didn't show and perceive any signs and symptoms or didn't feel anything odd in their bodies even at serum levels of above 200 milligrams/decilitre!

We started recording the sensitivity of patients towards raised blood sugar and calibrated or categorized in biochemistry quotient (short form: bio Q). So a person having serum levels of glucose 130 milligrams/decilitre who is feeling symptoms will have above-average biochemistry quotient than a person who is not feeling any symptom even if serum glucose levels are rocketing to 300 milligrams/ decilitre or more. In later cases, I'll say that the bio Q for that person will be very low for blood sugar.

The bio Q for a biochemistry test (criteria) x α perceived sensitivity to x.

x is any of the biochemistry tests serum levels in individuals.

This makes a lot of sense because assuming that we can reduce the threshold or increase sensitivity of perceived blood sugar levels in blood circulation, I have observed that they feel full earlier and even with low-glycaemic foods.

That led to *another discovery*: my weight management patients who had a lower threshold of serum glucose (in other words, more sensitive to rising blood glucose) were in the overweight category in comparison to low-glucose bio Q (high threshold for blood sugars or patients with less perceived sensitivity) and were all obese!

I would like to share a true story to support the relevance of blood sugar bio Q (biochemistry quotient). It's an interesting story.

I was a medical officer in the National Institute of Sports in 2009, and like most of you, I had a plan in my mind. I wanted to start my own weight loss clinic, so I resigned from my government job, and in that transition time, I bought a motorbike. Every alternate day, I used to go for a ride. My riding was mostly skill based, and I used to practise knee-down and fast riding skills. In medical terms, it is called learned motor coordination skills, and as you know, repetition is an important concept in motor learning. The more you practice, the better you get. New motor skills can be reinforced through practice in order to become stronger, more fluid, and more coordinated.

One day I noticed a strange thing in the morning when I went for a ride. I had a problem concentrating on my motor skills, and it was gross lack of concentration. Let me tell you that it was not my bad day at all. It happened again for two or three times in one month time, *but* I ignored it.

Being a doctor and scientist, I had to find an answer to this phenomenon rather than labelling it as just another bad day. This is what I found. I had high-glycaemic food at the night before every bad day. Then I did it deliberately for a couple of times, and finally, it became obvious to me that there was a strong connection between high-glycaemic foods and my fine motor coordination learning abilities.

To find a logical answer, I thought that my blood sugar might be going down after the spike from having high-glycaemic stuff. When you have high-sugar food, insulin is secreted by the pancreas to regulate it, and the insulin then causes the sugar level to reduce, which often overshoots, causing blood sugar levels below normal fasting levels.

So I thought of checking my blood sugar levels in those confused mornings, and nothing of that sort had happened. Rather, it was 110 milligrams/decilitre to 125 milligrams/decilitre every time I checked it on a non-concentration (unfocused) bad day, and I compared it to my good days of highest concentration with bike riding, where my blood sugar was around 75 to 85 milligrams/decilitre early in the morning.

Then my sister also noticed a similar pattern when she used to lift weights at the gym. After having simple carbohydrates, she was not able to concentrate that well. Later on, after a year of brainstorming, I had to figure it out. And that led me to devise a theory that could explain this phenomenon. And according to my theory, I had high bio Q for blood sugar as compared to a normal person. For me, 110 to 120 milligrams/decilitre of glucose levels will start giving symptoms of hyperglycaemia, and there is no other theory in the world that can explain this phenomenon of perceived symptoms for a given biochemical value, the theory that I call bio Q.

What I am telling you is a universal phenomenon and is just restricted to the bio Q of an individual person whether a person perceives the symptoms of hyperglycaemia at 110 or at 150 milligrams/decilitre. You can call this phenomenon as sugar brain fog, where the brain function blunts with rise in serum sugar levels.

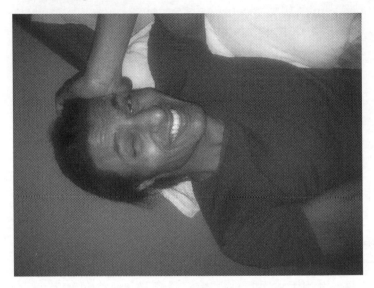

My idea of bio Q for blood sugar is the rating of perceived symptoms of hyperglycaemia at levels of, let's say, 120 milligrams/decilitre of blood glucose, which will have a bio Q of 120, and on the other extreme, a person who doesn't have any symptoms even at 200 milligrams/decilitre will have a bio Q of 40, as shown in tabulated form.

And a person who doesn't perceive any symptoms even at FBS 240 milligrams/decilitre and above, his or her bio Q will be 0. Just like lower IQ with lower marks in intelligence, you will give 0 to a person in terms of sensitivity to FBS.

Fasting Blood Sugar	Biochemistry Quotient
60	180
70	170
80	160
90	150
100	140
110	130
120	120
130	110
140	100
150	90
160	80
170	70
180	60
190	50
200	40
210	30
220	20
230	10
240	0
250	0
260	0

Like blood glucose, I have identified six more tests that qualify for determining biochemistry quotients in a person and they are.

Second Criterion: Uric Acid (Gout) Bio Q

The normal values for *uric acid* in females are 2 to 7 milligrams/decilitre, and for males, it's 2 to 8 milligrams/decilitre.

Excess of uric acid damages joints, especially the ankle and big toe (metatarsophalangeal joint). The problem here is the same. Some patients complain joint pains with all the signs and symptoms even at serum levels of uric acid as low as 6 milligrams/decilitre, and some of the patients don't even complain of any pain or any symptom even at levels as high as 10 milligrams/decilitre.

Obviously, people who have a lower threshold to serum uric acids will perceive higher levels of discomfort at relatively low levels of uric acid and will have much less chances of degeneration of the synovial joints because they are likely to adhere to the diet and medication recommended by doctors and are likely to be much healthier in the long term.

Almost 4 per cent of my overweight patients have a high uric acid biochemistry quotient, but there was no relation I could make that was directly relevant to weight gain. My criteria for uric acid bio Q 100 is when perceived symptoms, like pain and swelling, start with uric acid as low as 5 milligrams/decilitre.

And on the other extreme end of the spectrum, where the serum uric acid is at 10 milligrams/decilitre and above and still there is no symptom or joint pain, then you can say that the bio Q of that person is 0 for uric acid.

To calculate uric acid bio Q, you just have to match the value of serum uric acid in milligrams/decilitre where the patient starts feeling discomfort. At that value of bio Q, an example is of a patient who starts feeling discomfort at serum uric acid levels of 7 milligrams/decilitre; that person then has a bio Q of 60.

Uric acid (mg/dl)	Uric acid bio Q
5	100
6	80
7	60
8	40
9	20
10	0
>10	0

Third Criterion: Liver Function Test (ALT) Bio Q

Normal serum values of ALT (alanine aminotransferase) are between 5–45 units/litre for females, and for males, it's 7–56 units/litre.

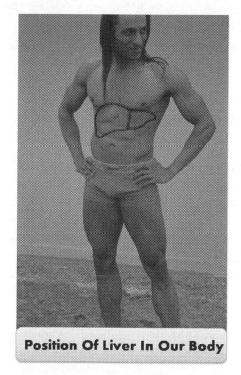

Position Of Liver In Our Body

Patients with higher bio Q for this test will have all the signs and symptoms of fatty liver despite ALT values being *around* the 45 units/litre range, and when we cure them for fatty liver, the response has been amazing. For patients who have a normal value and are symptomatic, I treat them as fatty-liver cases when they show most of the signs and symptoms of having fatty liver. If they show relevant history of intake of saturated animal fat, family history of gallstones, or a history of alcohol intake, I consider them as fatty liver cases and treat them on the same lines.

These are the patients who have a very low threshold of ALT. I have seen patients with values as low as 40 units/litre, showing signs and symptoms of fatty liver despite their ultrasound and bilirubin test being clean! Almost 20 per cent of my patients who come for weight loss complain of symptoms of fatty liver despite having a normal range of ALT.

If we use bio Q as one of the criteria for treating patients, then in my view, we can save future complications like gallstones before they even form.

Look at the immense possibilities of bio Q.

Just like the first two criteria, liver function bio Q is zero in people who don't have any symptoms of fatty liver but have ALT values of more than 150 units/litre, show grade II fatty liver in USG, and elevated bilirubin levels. And ask them what they feel or perceive in terms of symptoms or any signs, and they will say they do not perceive any symptoms. *Metabolic dumb* will be a harsh choice of words (you choose your term). And on the other side of the spectrum are the patients who have signs and symptoms of fatty liver and have fairly normal LFT. I call them bio Q genius.

I have noticed that almost 70 per cent of liver genius patients are not obese but are just overweight or came only for figure corrections. To know your patient's bio Q status, see the values against the serum values of ALT where your patient starts perceiving symptoms of fatty liver.

Liver function test (ALT) (U/L)	LFT bio Q
40	120
50	100
60	80
70	60
80	40
90	20
100	0
>100	0
>150	0
grade II fatty liver in USG	0

Fourth Criterion: Lipid Profile Bio Q

The normal ranges are:

- total cholesterol: 120–200 milligrams/decilitre
- HDL: 35–80 milligrams/decilitre for males and 40–80 milligrams/decilitre for females
- LDL: 80–110 milligrams/decilitre
- triglycerides: <150 milligrams/decilitre.

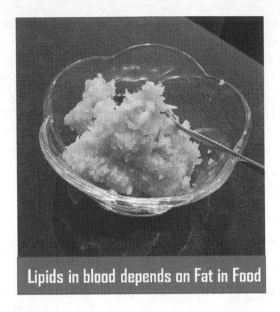

Lipids in blood depends on Fat in Food

Some patients show perceived signs and symptoms of increased cholesterol. Some people have reported strange sensations with increased cholesterol levels. Lately, I have found a fall in dyslipidemia in my patients. I am not sure of the exact reasons, but it might be that a lot of them were already on fibrates and related drugs before joining our weight loss therapies.

More studies need to be done on fresh cases. Most of my patients are from the urban population, and they all are obese. I am running a weight loss clinic, and 50 per cent of my patients are on medications for reducing cholesterol. I could detect cholesterol bio Q in only 5 per cent of the cases.

And trends were again similar, that bio Q genius patients needed only figure correction and, in some cases, were overweight but not obese.

Total cholesterol (mg/dl)	Cholesterol bio Q
150	100
160	90
170	80
180	70
190	60
200	50
210	40
220	30
230	20
240	10
250	0
>250	0

Fifth Criterion: Hydration Bio Q

Urinalysis usually consists of:

- blood urea nitrogen at 7–20 milligrams/decilitre
- creatinine at 0.7–1.1 milligrams/decilitre
- BUN–creatinine ratio at 5:35
- urine output.

We don't even have to do a biochemistry test to find dehydration in our patients. In my clinical experience, only 10 per cent of the patients are kidney bio Q geniuses. They are people who hydrate themselves well, and even a slight level of dehydration is well detected and felt by them. Unfortunately, 80 per cent of my patients have low kidney bio Q for hydration. Doctors are always scared of silent but life-threateningly serious, acute renal failure with no previous symptoms at all. But medical fraternity can be a great help if doctors evaluate kidney bio Q for every patient (just like U & E is done before any intervention or surgeries as standard operating procedure) as acute renal failure is the biggest threat in any surgical procedure.

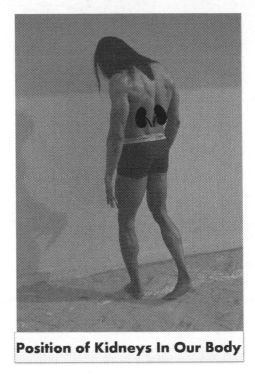

Position of Kidneys In Our Body

Microalbuminuria is a famous killer, especially in type 2 diabetes, which can be prevented by knowing the bio Q of a patient. Just for example, if the hydration bio Q is less in a person, then doctors can be more conscious of an underlying kidney problem that may occur in the future before giving any medication or surgical interventions.

To assess your hydration bio Q, just observe. When you start feeling thirsty, what is the percentage of total weight loss in a few hours?

Let's take my example here. If I go and do some workout in my gym, where the temperature and environmental conditions are constant throughout the year, I know that I start feeling thirsty when my body weight falls to about 1 per cent. My hydration bio Q according to the table will be 80, which is high, and I will replenish myself without dehydrating myself and thus avoiding undue stress on my kidneys.

This is just like my internal body asking for water, and I am not guided by external advice to have x number of glasses a day if my hydration bio Q is more.

On the other hand, if I know that my hydration bio Q is 30 or below, I should not depend upon my thirst mechanism or on my instincts and should replenish myself systematically by some external stimulus, like an alarm or reminder.

Body hydration (% weight reduction due to water loss)	Hydration bio Q
0.5	90
1	80
1.5	70
2	60
2.5	50
3	40
3.5	30
4	20
4.5	10
5	0
>5	0

Sixth Criterion: Blood Pressure Bio Q

The normal blood pressure is 120/80 to 140/90 depending on age.

Almost 80 per cent of my male obese patients are suffering from hypertension. Even in females, the figure is close to 50 per cent. I have already discussed about the recent data on hypertension done by AIIMS (All India Institute of Medical Sciences), India, where they found that 56 per cent of Indian urban females have hypertension.

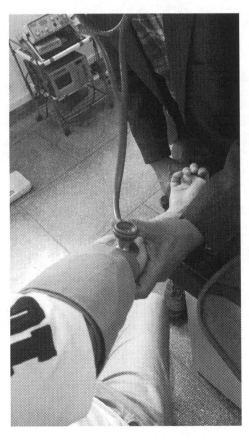

Ten per cent of my patients have high bio Q for blood pressure, and they start perceiving signs and symptoms of hypertension with blood pressure as low as 140/90.

And the other extremes are people who can't feel any abnormality even at high blood pressure of 180/110. If you make your patient aware that he or she is bio Q dumb for blood pressure, they should get their own BP apparatus for monitoring it or should frequently visit the doctor's clinic to get their blood pressure monitored regularly because they can't perceive it. Well, that makes a lot of sense in terms of treatment protocol.

To calculate the blood pressure bio Q, note down the systolic blood pressure of your patient when she or he starts feeling uneasy with the symptoms, and note down the bio Q. If the bio Q is high, the GP can tell the patient to go to them when they start feeling discomfort, and the patients who have low bio Q can be instructed not to follow their instincts but to rather come for regular check-ups or to keep track of their blood pressure regularly every day.

Systolic blood pressure (mm Hg)	Blood pressure bio Q
110	100
120	85
130	70
140	55
150	40
160	25
170	10
180	0
>180	0

Seventh Criterion: Hormone Imbalance

Thyroxine is my relevant hormone.

Thyroid bio Q	
T3 (total)	60–181 ng/ml
T4 (free)	0.8–1.5 ng/dl
T4 (total)	5.5–12.3 ng/ml
TBG	12–30 mg/l
Thyroid-stimulating hormone (TSH)	0.4–4.5 µIU/ml (normal values)

Increased TSH values and decreased T4 is hypothyroidism. Increased TSH and normal T4 happens in treated hypothyroidism or subclinical hypothyroidism.

Endocrinologists are quite divided in their opinions on when to start thyroxine treatment. Some start giving thyroxine when TSH levels rise above 8 micro international units/millilitre, and some start when values are 14 micro international units/millilitre and above. Many obese and overweight people think that they have hypothyroidism and that it's the cause of obesity, but when they are on thyroxine (hormone replacement therapy) and values of TSH, T3, and T4 are in normal range that they should start losing weight, that doesn't happen. At our clinic, 30 per cent of my female weight loss patients are undergoing treatment for hypothyroidism, and another 30 per cent have subclinical conditions.

The bio Q for thyroid function can be helpful in the treatment of a lot of obese patients. My patients with higher bio Q for thyroid function have all the symptoms of hypothyroidism despite TSH levels being as low as 3.5 micro international units/millilitre. Below that, I have kept it as a cut-off point. If TSH is between 3 and 5 micro international units/millilitre and the patient is showing some symptoms of hypothyroidism, I consider them as having genius bio Q and give them an aggressive diet (what we give to subclinical hypothyroid patients), and the results are good.

In cases of low bio Q for thyroid, patients don't feel many of the symptoms even if their TSH is skyrocketing at 25 or even 50! I had a female patient who was not showing any symptom typical of hypothyroid, and when we got her tests, her TSH was 152 micro international units/millilitre, and that is thyroid bio Q 0.

Thyroid-stimulating hormone (µIU/ml)	Thyroid Bio Q
3	100
3.5	90
4	80
4.5	70
5	60
5.5	50
6	40
6.5	30
7	20
7.5	10
8	0
>8	0

Eighth Criterion: Micronutrient Bio Q (Vitamins and Minerals)

I will be taking this topic in detail in my next book as this is a vast topic and this paragraph won't give justice to ergogenic supplements.

All I can say here is that my patients with genius micronutrient bio Q show the exact signs and symptoms of deficiency of a particular vitamin or mineral even if the serum levels are within range. And on the other end are patients on whom we get blood tests done and the serum levels will show exhausted micronutrients such as vitamin D and still no signs and symptoms were perceived by patients. I call it a micronutrient bio Q dumb condition.

Biochemistry Quotient's Relevance in Weight Loss

Among the eight biochemistry quotients, the most important ones that have a direct impact on weight management according to my observations are the liver, glucose, and thyroid bio Qs.

The higher your bio Q in these, the more your chances of being fit, and vice versa.

How Can You Use Bio Q in Clinical Practice?

The uses of bio Q can be many. My relevance is in obesity as that is the chronic disease of my interest.

- Real time e.g. of my patient Dr N. Kaur. In congruence of serum glucose and her perceived glucose, we found that she had a high bio Q for glucose. This information helped us to formulate a diet in which we could add high-GI food in her diet without worrying about overeating. Because of her low threshold for blood sugar, she used to feel full with a smaller quantity of food.

Now take the case of Mrs Vena (name changed), who had a blood sugar bio Q of 0. We stopped all high-glycaemic foods in her diet and told her to go for only sweeteners if she had sugar cravings and to have portions with proper measurements because her threshold for blood sugar was high. She didn't feel full even with higher quantities of food. And she was instructed to have low-glycaemic foods. So you see, the possibilities are virtually limitless.

- Similarly, we give customized diets to people who are specifically bio dumb for liver functions, hydration bio Q 0, thyroid functions, minerals and vitamins, uric acid bio Q 0, etc.

- Bio Q can be used for patients with any chronic disease. Doctors have to be strict and time-bound with patients who are bio Q dumb in specific biochemistry parameters and be liberal with patients who are geniuses in bio Q as they have a very good perceiving mechanism in the body so that they can intuitively take timely action when needed.

Now I hope you can see some science coming out of my theory and philosophy of bio Q!

Summary

1. I am defining biochemistry quotient (bio Q) as the ability of the body to perceive various biochemistry

measurements in plasma. The lower the threshold for perceiving (showing signs and symptoms), the higher the bio Q.

2. In relevance to obesity, I have chunked out eight bio Qs so that a doctor or scientist can easily grade a patient having genius, average, or dumb bio Q on the basis of blood tests and perceived signs and symptoms for that biochemistry measurement and seeing the charts to score their patients.

3. To weight managemet case relevance important bioQs are glucose bio Q, uric acid bio Q, liver bio Q, cholesterol bio Q, hydration bio Q, hormone bio Q, micronutrient bio Q.

4. There are limitless possibilities to customize a plan for your patient if you use this bio Q theory in relevant parameters. It can be drug dosages, diet plans, pre-operative and post-operative care, or anything that you can think of. The results can be promising, and the mortality rate can be lowered.

About the Author

Dr. Sunny Bawa is a sports doctor with a master's degree in sports medicine. He specializes in nutrition and micro-trauma injuries. He has an overall work experience of ten years of handling weight loss needs since 2006. He has been associated with athletes and games for so long. He was part of the *Doctors team for the 2010 Commonwealth Games in Delhi*. He has been the official team doctor for ICC World Cup, Indian Athletics (track and field team and boxing team).

A natural bodybuilder himself, he has won titles of Mr Mumbai and Mr Chandigarh. He still trains and coaches celebrities and pro athletes with special needs.

For further information, you can log on to:

www.nidsun.org

www.instagram.com/nidhimohankamal/

www.twitter.com/DrSunnyNidSun

The author has been in the weight management field since the year 2005 and has gifted new lives to thousands of people over this time.

One of the founders of NidSun clinics, he and his team has a vision to bring world-class health facilities to the common man at the best price, aiming for their long-term health-and-fitness goals, and hence provide quality lives free of diseases, which is the birthright of every human being.

NidSun is one of the first clinics in India to introduce cryolipolysis (fat-freezing procedure launched in 2013) and ultrasound fat blasting (launched in 2009), the best kind of weight loss anywhere in North India. NidSun Weight Loss is a pioneer in these treatments and have successfully treated thousands of clients seeking body shaping in Delhi, Chandigarh, and the rest of North India. Thousands of people have benefited from the packages and continue to maintain them till date.

The NidSun clinic came to existence as a result of the combined efforts of Dr Sunny Bawa and Nidhi Mohan Kamal (his sister) in 2007. The team has now grown bigger and includes an energetic team of doctors, dieticians, nutrition experts, physiologists, counsellors, trainers, and top-notch hospitality staff and therapists.

NidSun Weight Loss *aims to provide, serve, and help people come out of lifestyle-related ailments related to overweight.*

The people are NidSun's greatest assets and biggest differentiators. The NidSun Weight Loss staff is passionate about results and are ambitious and impatient for success.

Printed in the United States
By Bookmasters